Student Hand

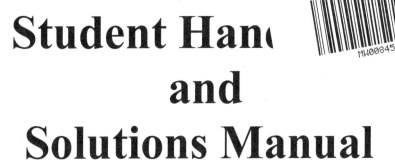

and
Solutions Manual

Essentials of Genetics
TENTH EDITION

Harry Nickla

Professor Emeritus, Creighton University

Michelle F. Gaudette

Lecturer Emerita, Tufts University

William S. Klug

College of New Jersey

Michael R. Cummings

Illinois Institute of Technology

Charlotte A. Spencer

University of Alberta

Michael A. Palladino

Monmouth University

Darrell J. Killian

Colorado College

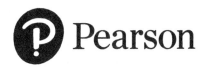 Pearson

Courseware Portfolio Manager: Michael Gillespie
Director of Portfolio Management: Beth Wilbur
Courseware Director, Content Development: Ginnie Simione Jutson
Courseware Portfolio Management Assistant: Ashley Fallon
Managing Producer: Michael Early
Product Marketing Manager: Alysun Estes
Rich Media Content Producer: Robert Johnson
Full-Service Vendor: SPi Global
Content Producer: Brett Coker, SPi Global
Full-Service Editorial Project Manager: Dinesh Deivendiran, SPi Global
Illustrations: Cenveo Publishing Services and SPi Global
Cover and Interior Printer: LSC Communications
Manufacturing Buyer: Stacey J. Weinberger
Cover Photo: Andrew Syred / Science Source

ISBN 10: **0-135-30042-8**; ISBN 13: **978-0-135-30042-8**

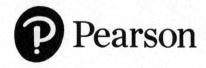

www.pearson.com

Contents

Students, Read This Section First

How to Increase Your Chances of Success in Genetics:

1. Attend Class
2. Read the Book
3. Do the Assigned Problems
4. Don't Cram
5. Study When There Are No Tests
6. Develop Confidence from Effort
7. Set Disciplined Study Goals
8. Learn Concepts
9. Be Careful with Old Exams
10. Don't "Second Guess" the Teacher

A first course in genetics can be a humbling experience for many students. The intent of this book is to help you understand introductory genetics as presented in the text **Essentials of Genetics** (10th edition). It is possible that the lowest grades received in one's major, or even in one's undergraduate career, may be in genetics. Don't let this discourage you – you are not alone. I have known successful geneticist for whom college-level genetics did not come easily at first. When this happens, it is not unusual for some students to become frustrated with their own seeming inability to succeed in genetics. This frustration is felt by teachers as they field the following types of student comments:

"I studied all the material but failed your test."

"I must have a mental block to it. I just don't get it. I just don't understand what you are asking."

"Where did you get that question? I didn't see anything like that in the book or in my notes."

"This is the first test I have **ever** failed."

"I helped three of my friends last night and I got the lowest grade."

"I am getting a 'D' in your course and I have never received less than a 'B' in my whole life."

"I stayed up all night studying for your exam and I still failed."

Similar to Algebra

Think back to the first time you encountered "word problems" in your first algebra class. How many times did you ask yourself, your parents, or your teacher the following classic question?

> "I hate word problems, I just can't understand them, and why do I need to learn this anyway, I'll never use it?"

At that time, you had two choices: give in to your frustrations and be afraid of problem solving for the rest of your life (which, unfortunately, happens too often) or regroup, seek help, strip away distractions, and focus on learning something new and powerful. Because you are taking genetics, you probably succeeded in algebra, perhaps with difficulty at first, and you will probably succeed in genetics.

In algebra, you were forced to convert something real and dynamic (e.g., two trains leaving at different times from different stations at different speeds) to a somewhat abstract formula that can be applied to an infinite number of similar problems. In genetics you will again learn something new. It will involve the conversion of something real and dynamic (genes, chromosomes, hereditary elements, gamete formation, gene splicing, and evolution) to an array of general concepts (similar to mathematical formulas) that will allow you to predict the outcome of an infinite number of presently known and yet-to-be-discovered phenomena relating to the origin and maintenance of life.

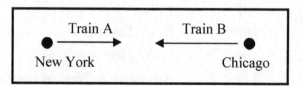

Students, Read This Section First

Mental Pictures and Symbols

When working almost any word problem, it is often helpful to make a simple drawing that relates, in space, the primary participants. From that drawing one can often predict or estimate a likely outcome. A mathematical formula and its solution provide a precise outcome. To understand genetics, it is often helpful to make drawings of the participants, whether they be crosses ($Aa \times Aa$), gametes (A or a), or molecules (anticodon interacting with codon).

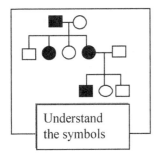

As with algebra, symbols used to represent a multitude of structures, movements, and interactions are abstract, informative, and fundamental to understanding the discipline. It is the set of symbols and their interrelationships that comprise the concepts that make up the framework of genetics. Test questions and problems exemplify the concepts and may be completely unfamiliar to the student; nevertheless, they refer directly to the basic concepts of genetics.

Attendance and Attention Are Mandatory

Many professors do not take attendance in lectures; therefore, it is likely that some students will opt to take a day off now and then. While this might seem harmless, remember that learning is cumulative. Concepts presented in each class will be essential to understanding concepts presented later in the course. In general, continual absences will usually result in confusion and failure.

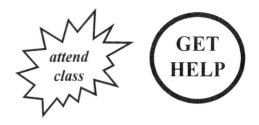

Recall how challenging it was to set up and understand the first algebra word problem on your own. It is likely that your ultimate source of understanding came from the course instructor. Although using the text is important in your understanding of genetics, the teacher can walk you through the concepts and strategies much more efficiently than a text because a text is organized in a sequential manner. A good teacher can "cut and paste" an idea from here and there as needed.

To benefit from the wisdom of the instructor, the student must concentrate and listen actively during the lecture session rather than sit, passively, assuming that the ideas can be figured out at a later date. Taking notes is a good start to active listening. *Thinking about* the material as you take notes, and *reviewing* the material *soon after it was presented* should also help in solidifying concepts. In addition, the instructor will not be able to cover all the material in the text. Parts will be emphasized, whereas other areas may be omitted entirely.

There is no magic formula for understanding genetics or any other discipline of significance. Learning anything, especially at the college level, requires time, patience, and confidence. A student must be willing to focus on the subject matter for an hour or so *each day* over the entire semester (quarter, trimester, etc.). Study time must be free of distractions and pressured by realistic goals.

The student must be patient and disciplined, studying even when no assignments are due and no tests are looming.

Because it is the instructor who writes and grades the tests, who is in a better position to prepare the students for those tests?

The majority of successful students are willing to read the text ahead of the lecture material, spend time thinking about the concepts and examples, and work as many sample problems as possible. They study for a period of time, stop, then return to review the most difficult areas. They do not try to cram information into marathon study sessions a few nights before the examinations. Although some may get away with that practice on occasion, more often than not, understanding the concepts in genetics requires more mature study habits and preparation.

Perhaps a Different Way of Thinking

Because the acquisition of problem-solving ability requires that students rely on new and important ways of seeing things rather than memorizing the book and notes, some students find the transition more challenging than others. Some students are more able to deal in the abstract, concept-oriented framework than others. Students who have typically relied on "pure memorization" for their success will find a need to focus on concepts and 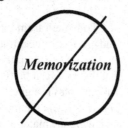 problem solving. They may struggle at first, just as they may have struggled with the first word problem in algebra. There is, and should be, a healthy conflict between the student and a challenging teacher. The reward for such conflict is intellectual growth. That's what college is supposed to stimulate. With such growth will come an increased ability to solve a variety of problems beyond genetics. Problem solving is a process, a style, that can be applied to many disciplines. Few people are actually born with the touch of synthetic brilliance. Success comes from probing deeply into a few areas to see how problems are approached in a given discipline. Then, because problems are usually approached in a fairly consistent manner, a given problem-solving approach can often be applied to a variety of activities.

Read ahead. You have likely been told that it is important to read the assigned material before attending lectures. This allows you to make full use of the information provided in the lecture and to concentrate on those areas that are unclear in the readings. If the concept is still unclear during or after the lecture, your preparation should allow you to ask more focused questions. By recognizing what you *do* understand, you can ask for clarification of a particular point that is still unclear. It is very likely that your question will be quickly dealt with to your

benefit and the benefit of others in the class. If you do not have the opportunity to ask questions in class, or if you are still unsure of what your question is, revisit the text and your notes. Consider your questions for a day or two and if not resolved, schedule an appointment with the instructor. Obviously, cramming for examinations does not allow for such a mature approach to study.

> ## Ask Questions
> ## and
> ## Don't Tune Out!

How to Study

Genetics is a science that involves symbols (A, b, p), structures (chromosomes, ribosomes, plasmids), and processes (meiosis, replication, translation) that interact in a variety of ways. Models describe the manner in which hereditary units are made, how they function, and how they are transmitted from parent to offspring. Because many parts of the models interact in both time and space, genetics can not be viewed as a discipline filled with facts that should be memorized. Rather, one must be, or become, comfortable with seeking to understand both the components of the models as well as the way the models work.

One can memorize the names and shapes of all the parts of an automobile engine, but without studying the interrelationships among the parts in time and space, one will have little understanding of the real nature of the engine. It takes time, work, and patience to see how an engine works, and it will take time, work, and patience to understand genetics.

> ## Time,
> ## Work,
> ## Patience

Don't cram. A successful tennis player doesn't learn to play tennis overnight; therefore, you can't expect to learn genetics under the pressure of night-long cramming. It will be necessary for you to develop and follow a realistic study schedule for genetics as well as for the other courses you are taking. It is important that you focus your study periods into intensive but short sessions each day throughout the entire

> ## Study when
> ## there are
> ## no tests.

semester (quarter, trimester). Because genetics tests often require you to think "on the spot," it is very important that you get a good night's sleep before each test. Avoid caffeine in the evening before the test because a clear, rested, well-prepared mind will be required.

Study goals. The instruction of genetics is often divided into large conceptual units, and one unit builds toward the next. A test usually follows each unit, but should not be seen as an end-point: mastery of an early unit is almost always required for success in later units. It will be necessary for you to study genetics on a routine basis long before each test and to retain your understanding of this material throughout (and beyond!) the course. To do so, set specific study goals and adhere to them. Don't let examinations in one course interfere with the study goals of another course. Notice that each course being taken is handled in the same way—study ahead of time and don't cram.

There are a number of different study strategies that students use. One favored by many instructors is group learning. Forming a study group that meets on a regular basis can be quite helpful in reinforcing your understanding of the concepts and applications taught. Group members can talk each other through the steps of complex processes – and point out if one member skips a step or does not explain a step thoroughly. Group members can also work through some suggested problems together (but **not** graded, assigned problems, unless the instructor grants permission to do so). However, do not become dependent on the group – you need to be able to reason through concepts and problem solving on your own.

If you find group learning unappealing, try speaking aloud while studying and solving problems. As you explain the steps to yourself, you may reach a point where you cannot find the "right words" to express yourself. Don't dismiss this as a fluke, because you are sure you understand. Instead, see this as an indication that you are not entirely clear on the concept and need to review or to seek help from your instructor.

Study each subject at least every other day—especially when there are no tests!

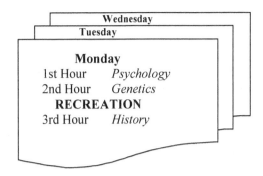

Develop a Realistic Monthly Schedule

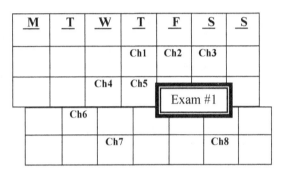

Develop a Plan for the Semester

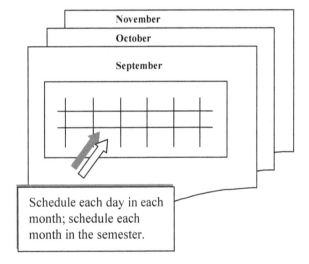

Schedule each day in each month; schedule each month in the semester.

Too much? If the above scheduling seems like overkill, remember that you and/or someone else made significant sacrifices for you to attend college. Make the most of it and realize that, more than likely, you will only have one period in your life to get this right.

Work the assigned problems. The basic concepts of genetics are generally straightforward, but there are many examples that apply to these concepts. To help students adjust to the variety of examples and approaches to concepts, instructors often assign practice problems from the back of each chapter. If your instructor has assigned certain problems, finish working them as close to the assignment date as possible, but *no later than* one week before each examination. Before starting a set of problems, read the chapter carefully and consider the information presented in class.

Suggestions for working problems:

(1) Work the problem without looking at the answer. Commit each answer to paper!

(2) Check your answer in this book.

(3) If incorrect, work the problem again.

(4) If still incorrect, you don't understand the concept.

(5) Reread your lecture notes and the text.

(6) Work the problem again.

(7) If you still don't understand the solution, mark it, and go to the next problem.

In your next study session, return to those problems that you have marked. Expect to make mistakes and learn from those mistakes. Sometimes what is difficult to see one day may be obvious the next. If you are still having problems with a concept, schedule a meeting with your instructor. Usually the problem can be cleared up in a few minutes. Be sure to go back and try to solve these problems again, to verify your understanding.

You will notice that in this book, we have presented the solution to each problem. We provide

different ways of looking at some of the problems. Instructors often take a problem directly from those at the end of the chapters or they will modify an existing problem. Reversing the "direction" of a question is a common approach. Instead of giving characteristics of the parents and asking for characteristics of the offspring, the question may provide characteristics of the offspring and ask for particulars on the parents. Think as you work the problems.

Separate examples from concepts. As mentioned earlier, genetics boils down to a few basic concepts. However, there are many examples that apply those concepts. Too often, students have trouble separating examples from the concepts. Examples allow you to picture, in concrete terms, various phenomena, but they don't exemplify each phenomenon or concept in its entirety.

Be careful when using old examinations. Often it is customary for students to have access to old examinations. While this can provide students with additional practice problems or the opportunity for a "dry run" of the exam, there are also

---

Old examinations may help, but...

---

disadvantages. A **good** use of old examinations is as a "practice," taken under examination conditions (timed, in a quiet space where you will not be interrupted and do not have access to texts or a computer). You should "grade" the examination stringently and review concepts missed. However, be aware that using "practice examinations" can be loaded with pitfalls. First, students often, albeit unconsciously, find themselves "second guessing" questions on an upcoming examination. They forget that an examination usually only covers a subset of the available information in a section. Therefore, entire conceptual areas may have been presented that have not appeared on recent exams.

Also, material taught in previous years may have been presented in less detail than in the current year, so a correct answer on an old examination may not be acceptable for the current year. In addition, if a question has the same general structure as one on a previous examination but is modified on the current examination, students often provide an answer for the "old" question rather than the one being asked. Granted, it is of value to see the format of each question and the general emphasis of previous examinations, but remember that each examination is potentially a new production capable of covering areas that have not been tested before. This is especially likely in a course such as genetics where the material changes very rapidly.

> *Don't try to figure out what will be asked.*
> *Study all the material as well as possible.*

Structure of This Book

The intent of this book is to help you understand the concepts of genetics as given in the text and most likely given in the lectures, then to apply these concepts to the solution of all problems and questions at the end of each chapter. Rather than merely providing you with the solutions to the problems, we have tried to walk you through each component of most questions so that you can see from where information is obtained and how it can be applied in the solution. At the beginning of each chapter is a section that relates general concept areas being tested to particular problems. This should help you practice certain conceptual areas as needed without necessarily having to work every single problem at the end of each chapter.

> **Master each listed term, its context, and related examples.**

Listing of terms, structures, and concepts. Understanding the vocabulary of a discipline is essential to understanding the discipline. Throughout the text by Klug et al. you will find terms in bold print. Those words, plus others, have been listed at the front of each chapter in this handbook. In some cases, certain terms are identified (*) that deserve special attention. Be certain to master an understanding of each listed term as to its precise meaning, the context in which it is presented, and examples relating to each.

Use the listings as checklists to make certain that you understand the meaning of each term in each chapter. Notice that the various terms are not redefined in this handbook, so it is important that you use the text for the original definitions.

> **Understand the words and phrases of the discipline.**

Solved problems and discussion questions. Each of the problems at the end of each chapter is solved from a beginner's point of view. Some of the answers to the questions and problems will refer you to the textbook. Be certain that you fully understand the solution to each of the questions suggested or assigned by your instructor. Consider also that the same concept (question) can be addressed in a variety of ways. Try to anticipate a variety of approaches to the same concept (question).

DEDICATION

We dedicate this edition to our long-time colleague and friend, Harry Nickla, who sadly passed away in 2017. With decades of experience teaching Genetics to students at Creighton University, Harry's contribution to our texts included authorship of this *Student Handbook and Solutions Manual* and the text bank, as well as devising some of the problems at the end of each chapter. He was also a source of advice during the planning session for each new edition, and during our many revisions. We always appreciated his professional insights, friendship, and conviviality. We were lucky to have him as part of our team, and we miss him greatly.

WSK, MRC, CAS, MAP, DJK, and MFG.

Chapter 1: Introduction to Genetics

Concept Areas	Corresponding Problems
Mendelism	1, 3, 4
Homologous Chromosomes	4
Chromosome Theory of Inheritance	3, 6
Central Dogma of Molecular Biology	5, 6, 7, 8
Molecular Biology	2, 8, 9, 10, 11
Genetics and Social Issues	12, 13, 14, 15, 16
Model Organisms	14

Structures and Processes Checklist—Significant items that deserve special attention are identified with a "*".

(Check topic when mastered–provide examples where appropriate–understand the context of each entry)

- **Overview**

  - CRISPR-Cas*

  - gene editing*

  - "seek and destroy" mechanism

- **Early History of Genetics**

  - Aristotle, 350 B.C.

  - William Harvey, 1600s

  - epigenesis*

  - preformationism

  - homunculus

  - Matthias Schleiden, Theodor Schwann, 1830

  - cell theory*

  - spontaneous generation

  - Louis Pasteur

  - Charles Darwin, 1859

  - evolution*

  - natural selection*

  - Gregor Mendel, 1866

  - Carl Correns, Hugo de Vries, Erich Tschermak, 1900

- **From Mendel to DNA**

  - genetics*

  - diploid number ($2n$)*

  - homologous chromosomes*

  - cell division

  - mitosis

  - meiosis*

  - haploid number (n)*

  - Sutton, Boveri

  - chromosome theory of inheritance*

  - genetic variation*

  - mutation*

- allele*
- phenotype*
- genotype*
- DNA or protein*
- Avery, MacLeod, McCarty, 1944
- DNA carries genetic information*
- Hershey, Chase

- **Molecular Genetics**

  - Watson, Crick, 1953
  - nucleotides (ATGC)*
  - Wilkins, Watson, Crick, 1962
  - transcription*
  - messenger RNA (mRNA)
  - ribosome
  - translation*
  - genetic code*
  - codon*
  - transfer RNA (tRNA)
  - diversity of proteins and biological functions*
  - 20 amino acids
  - enzymes
  - hemoglobin
  - linking genotype to phenotype*
  - sickle-cell anemia
  - central dogma of molecular biology*

- **DNA Cloning**

  - restriction enzyme*

- vectors
- clones
- genome
- library
- recombinant DNA technology*

- **Expanding Impact of Biotechnology**

  - biotechnology*
  - transgenic organisms*
  - cloned organisms*
  - therapeutic proteins
  - genetic testing

- **Genomics, Proteomics, and Bioinformatics**

  - Human Genome Project (HGP)
  - genomics*
  - proteomics*
  - bioinformatics*
  - classical or forward genetics
  - reverse genetics
  - gene knockout*

- **Genetics and Model Organisms**

  - model organisms*
  - classical genetics studies
  - developmental studies
  - models of human disease

- **Societal Impact**

  - Nobel Prizes
  - ethics and oversight

2

F1.1 Simple diagram of the central dogma of molecular genetics, showing the flow of information in cells

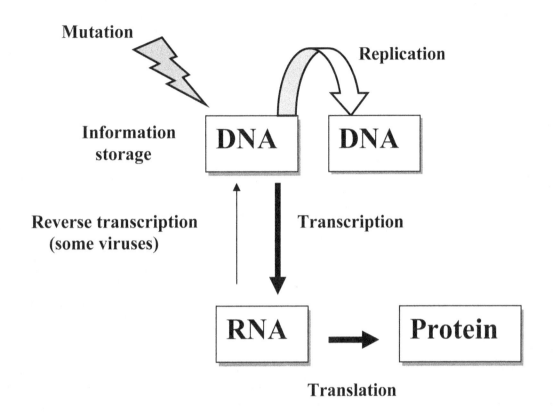

Chapter 1 Introduction to Genetics

Solutions to Problems and Discussion Questions

1. Mendel proposed that traits are passed from one generation to the next by following certain predictable patterns. He hypothesized that traits in peas are controlled by discrete units, which are now called genes. He also suggested that these units occur in pairs and that the members of each gene pair separate from each other during gamete formation.

2. Your essay should include a description of the impact of recombinant DNA technology on the following: plant and animal husbandry and production, drug development, medical advances, and understanding of gene function.

3. The chromosome theory of inheritance states that inherited traits are controlled by genes residing on chromosomes, which are transmitted by gametes. The behavior of chromosomes parallels Mendel's model of heredity, providing a mechanism for Mendel's observed results.

4. A gene variant is called an allele. There can be many such variants in a population, but a diploid individual can have a maximum of only two such alleles for any given gene. The genotype of an organism is defined as the specific allelic or genetic constitution of an organism; often the allelic composition of one or a limited number of genes is being considered. The observable sum of features of those genes is called the phenotype.

5. At the time, it was known that proteins consist of amino acids, and 20 structurally and chemically unique subunits had been identified. By contrast, DNA was known to consist of only six different components (sugar, phosphate, and four nitrogenous bases) arranged in a linear fashion. Genes were known to encode and control a variety of functions; therefore, it seemed reasonable that the genetic material should be abundant and versatile. DNA was considered neither complex nor versatile because of its limited variety of subunits. Proteins, however, were seen as capable of providing a vast amount of functional variation due to the rich variety of subunits available. Therefore, proteins were considered more likely to be the genetic material.

6. *Genes* are the functional units of heredity. They consist of linear sequences of nucleotides and usually exert their influence by producing proteins through the processes of transcription and translation.

Chromosomes are long double strands of complementary nucleotides that contain linear assemblies of genes. In many organisms, nucleotides associate with specific proteins. Chromosomes (and by extension, genes) are duplicated by a variety of enzymes so that daughter cells inherit complete copies of the parental hereditary information.

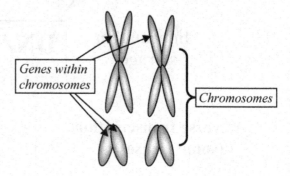

7. Genetic information is encoded in DNA by the sequence of bases. This sequence is transcribed into messenger RNA products, which are then translated into proteins.

8. The central dogma of molecular genetics refers to the relationships among DNA, RNA, and proteins. The processes of *transcription* and *translation* are integral to understanding these relationships. (See F1.1 in this handbook.) DNA stores the genetic information and serves as the template for its own reproduction (replication) and for the production of RNA copies (transcription). RNA, in turn, carries this information to be used for the synthesis of proteins (translation). Because DNA and RNA are discrete chemical entities, they can be isolated, studied, and manipulated in a variety of experiments that define modern genetics.

9. For any protein chain, each position is filled by one of 20 amino acids. The total number of possible combinations is the mathematical product of the possibilities at each position. So, if a protein chain is 5 amino acids long, there would be $20 \times 20 \times 20 \times 20 \times 20$ (or 20^5) different possible combinations. As the length of an amino acid chain increases, the number of possible combinations becomes very large.

10. Restriction enzymes (endonucleases) cut double-stranded DNA at particular base sequences. Vectors are carrier DNA molecules that can enter and replicate in cells. When vector and target DNAs are cleaved with the same enzyme, complementary ends are created, which can be combined and ligated (sealed together) to form intact double-stranded structures. Once recombinant molecules enter bacterial cells, they can replicate, producing many copies or clones.

11. In the past 40 years, traditional transmission, cytological, and molecular genetics have provided an understanding of many aspects of both plant and animal biology, including development of pest-resistant crops and identification of hazardous organisms in our food (*E. coli,* for example). Recently, biotechnology has allowed genes to be moved in a variety of ways to generate transgenic plants. Such plants can be engineered to increase their ecological breadth, disease resistance, and/or nutrient value. Wheat, rice, corn, and beans are among the crops that have been modified.

12. Unique transgenic plants and animals can be patented, as ruled by the U.S. Supreme Court in 1980. Supporters of organismic patenting argue that it is needed to encourage innovation and allow the costs of discovery to be recovered. Capital investors assume that it is likely that their investments will yield positive returns. Others argue that natural substances should not be privately owned, and that, once owned by a small number of companies, free enterprise will be stifled. Individuals and companies needing vital but patented products may have limited access. Such concentration of products might reduce genetic variation because farmers will be forced to grow a limited suite of crops.

13. It can be argued that some mechanism, such as patents, should be in place to protect the investments of individuals and institutions that develop needed and useful products, such as selected stretches of human DNA. However, safeguards, both ethical and economic, need to be developed to ensure that relatively free and fair access exists when vital issues are in question. Any mechanism needs to protect both investors and consumers.

14. Model organisms are not only useful, but also necessary for understanding genes that influence human diseases. Given that genetic/molecular systems are highly conserved across broad phylogenetic lines, what is learned in one organism can usually be applied to many other organisms. In addition, most model organisms have useful characteristics, such as ease of growth, genetic understanding, or abundant offspring, that make them straightforward and especially informative in genetic studies.

15. This question is open to a variety of answers, depending on the individual. Although it may be difficult to put yourself in this position, consider not only what your decision would be, but also why you would make such a decision. Often, as a person ages, his or her perspective changes; for example, the possibility of having children and passing the disease allele to them might have a stronger influence on your decision at a younger age than at an older age. Conversely, quality of life issues might weigh more heavily as you age.

16. For approximately 60 years, discoveries in genetics have guided our understanding of living systems, aided rational drug design, and dominated many social discussions. Genetics provides the framework for universal biological processes and helps explain species stability and diversity. Given the central focus of genetics in so many of life's processes, it is understandable why so many genetic scientists have been awarded the Nobel Prize.

Chapter 2: Mitosis and Meiosis

Concept Areas	Corresponding Problems
Cell Structure	3
Homology of Chromosomes	1, 4, 5, 12, 23
Cell Division	1, 2, 7, 8, 9, 13
Mitosis	2, 6, 8, 9, 12, 14, 15, 19, 25, 30
Meiosis	2, 9, 10, 11, 12, 13, 14, 15, 16, 17, 18, 19, 20, 24, 26, 27, 28, 29, 30
Chromosome Structure	1, 4, 5, 7, 19, 21, 22, 23

Structures and Processes Checklist—Significant items that deserve special attention are identified with a "*".

(Check topic when mastered–provide examples where appropriate–understand the context of each entry)

- **Overview**
  - chromosomes
  - mitosis*
  - meiosis*
  - gametes or spores
  - chromatin
- **Cell Structure**
  - plasma membrane
  - cell wall
  - glycocalyx, or cell coat
  - receptor molecules
  - eukaryotes*
  - nucleus
  - nucleolus
  - nucleolus organizer region (NOR)
  - prokaryotes*
  - nucleoid
  - cytoplasm
  - cytosol
  - cytoskeleton
  - endoplasmic reticulum (ER)
  - ribosomes*
  - mitochondria*
  - chloroplasts
  - centrioles
  - centrosome
  - spindle fibers
- **Chromosomes***
  - centromere
  - metacentric
  - submetacentric
  - acrocentric

6

- telocentric
- centromere
- p arm, q arm
- diploid number (2*n*)*
- homologous chromosomes*
- karyotype
- haploid number (*n*)*
- genome
- locus (pl. loci)
- biparental inheritance
- alleles*
- sex-determining chromosomes
- **Mitosis Partitions Chromosomes***
  - zygotes
  - karyokinesis
  - cytokinesis
  - cell cycle
  - interphase*
  - S phase*
  - G1 (gap I)*
  - G2 (gap II)*
  - DNA replication*
  - M phase*
  - G0 stage
  - prophase
  - sister chromatids*
  - cohesin
  - equatorial plane, or metaphase plate
  - prometaphase

- metaphase*
- kinetochore
- separase
- shugoshin
- kinetochore microtubules
- anaphase*
- disjunction
- daughter chromosome
- telophase*
- cytokinesis
- cell plate
- middle lamella
- cell furrow
- transition to interphase
- control of cell cycle*
- *cell division cycle* (*cdc*) mutations*
- kinases
- cyclins
- cyclin-dependent kinases
- cell-cycle checkpoints*
- potential malignancy*
- **Meiosis Creates Haploid Gametes***
  - meiosis*
  - genetic continuity
  - genetic variation
  - crossing over*
  - prophase I*
  - sister chromatids*
  - synapsis*

- bivalent*
- tetrad*
- chiasma (pl. chiasmata)*
- nonsister chromatids*
- metaphase I*
- random alignment*
- anaphase I*
- dyad*
- disjunction*
- nondisjunction*
- telophase I*
- second meiotic division*
- meiosis II*
- prophase II*
- metaphase II*
- anaphase II*
- telophase II*
- monad*
- haploid state*
- **Development of Gametes***
  - spermatogenesis*
  - spermatogonium*
  - primary spermatocyte*

- secondary spermatocyte*
- spermatid*
- spermiogenesis
- spermatozoa, or sperm
- oogenesis*
- ovum (pl. ova)
- primary oocyte*
- oogonium*
- first polar body*
- secondary oocyte*
- ootid*
- second polar body*
- **Meiosis and Sexual Reproduction***
  - diploid organisms*
  - diploid to haploid
  - genetic variation*
  - sporophyte stage
  - gametophyte stage
  - alternation of generations*
- **Electron Microscopy**
  - histones
  - folded-fiber model
  - 5000-fold compaction

F2.1 Diagram illustrating the stages of interphase. Also shown are chromosome number and structure in an organism with a diploid chromosome number of 4 ($2n = 4$). Individual chromosomes cannot be seen at interphase; therefore, the chromosomes pictured here are hypothetical and intended to indicate that chromosome number does not change even though the DNA content doubles during the S phase. Notice that the chromosomes are doubled structures in the G2 phase.

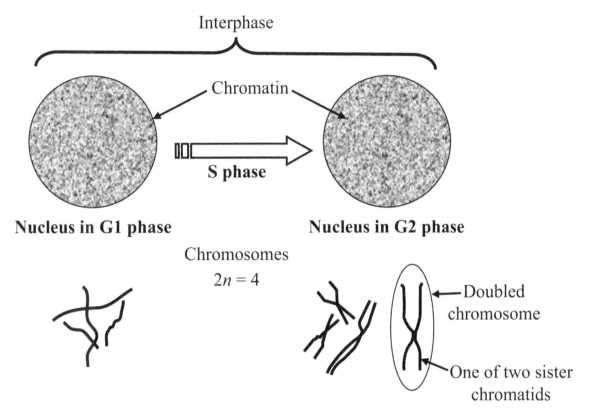

F2.2 Important nomenclature referring to chromosomes and associated genes. Shown below are metaphase I chromosomes in an organism where the diploid chromosome number is 4 ($2n = 4$). There are two pairs of chromosomes: one pair is large and metacentric, and the second is small and telocentric. Sister chromatids are identical to each other because they result from DNA replication of a chromosome, whereas homologous chromosomes are chromosomes of the same type and are similar to each other in terms of overall size, centromere location, function, gene location, and other factors described in the text.

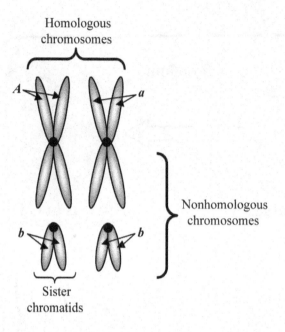

F2.3 Illustration of chromosomes of mitotic cells in an organism with a chromosome number of 4 ($2n = 4$).

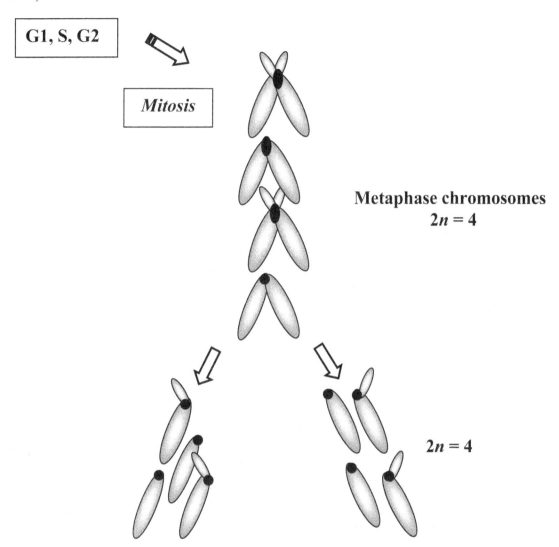

F2.4 Illustration of chromosomes of meiotic cells in an organism with a chromosome number of 4 ($2n = 4$).

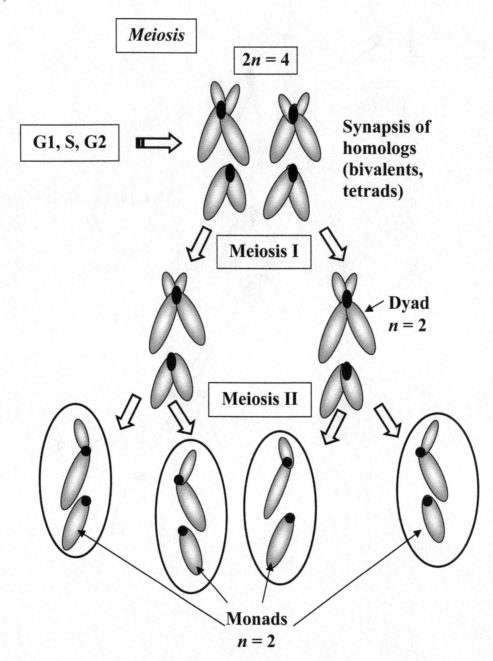

Answers to Now Solve This

2.1 (a) The first sentence tells you that $2n = 16$ and that it is a question about mitosis. Because each chromosome in prophase is doubled (having gone through an S phase) and is visible at the end of prophase, there should be 32 chromatids. Refer to F2.3 in this handbook to see an example with $2n = 4$. Notice that there are four doubled chromosomes in prophase, so there are eight chromatids visible at late prophase.

(b) Because the centromeres divide and what were previously sister chromatids migrate to opposite poles during anaphase, there should be 16 daughter chromosomes moving to each pole.

2.2 Look carefully at F2.4 in this handbook and notice that for a diploid cell with four chromosomes, there are two tetrads each composed of a homologous pair of chromosomes.

(a) If there are 16 chromosomes (8 pairs of homologous chromosomes), there should be eight tetrads.

(b) After meiosis I and in the second meiotic prophase, there are as many dyads as there are pairs of chromosomes. There will be eight dyads.

(c) Because the monads migrate to opposite poles during meiosis II (from the separation of dyads), there should be eight monads migrating to *each* pole.

2.3 The genotype of the second polar body will not necessarily be identical to that of the ootid. If crossing over occurs during meiosis I, then the chromatids in the secondary oocyte will not be identical. Once the chromatids of each chromosome separate during meiosis II, dissimilar chromatids reside in the ootid and the second polar body.

Chapter 2 Mitosis and Meiosis

Solutions to Problems and Discussion Questions

1. (a) Examination of karyotypes of somatic cells from the same species shows they contain the same number of chromosomes. The lengths, centromere placements, and banding patterns of nearly all such chromosomes can be matched into pairs.

(b) The initiation and completion of DNA synthesis can be detected by the incorporation of labeled precursors into DNA. DNA content in a G2 nucleus is twice that of a G1 nucleus.

(c) During interphase, the nucleus is filled with chromatin fibers. These disappear (and condensed chromosomes appear) during mitosis. Electron microscopic observations indicate that mitotic chromosomes are in varying states of extensively folded structures derived from chromatin.

2. Mitosis maintains chromosomal constancy, so there is no change in chromosome number or kind in the two daughter cells. By contrast, meiosis provides for a reduction in chromosome number and an opportunity for exchange of genetic material between homologous chromosomes. This leads to the production of numerous potentially different haploid (*n*) cells. During oogenesis, only one of the four meiotic products is functional; however, four of the four meiotic products of spermatogenesis are potentially functional. Errors during either mitosis or meiosis (such as nondisjunction events) can lead to cells with too many or too few chromosomes.

3. (a) *Chromatin* contains the genetic material that is responsible for maintaining hereditary information (from one cell to daughter cells and from one generation to the next) and production of the phenotype. During interphase of the cell cycle (mitotic and meiotic), chromosomes are not condensed and are in a genetically active, spread out form (chromatin). In this condition, chromosomes are not visible as individual structures under the microscope (light or electron). See F2.1 for a sketch of what chromatin might look like.

(b) The *nucleolus* (pl. *nucleoli*) is a structure that is produced by activity of the nucleolus organizer region in eukaryotes. Composed of ribosomal DNA and protein, it is the structure for the production of ribosomes. Some nuclei have more than one nucleolus. Nucleoli are not present during mitosis or meiosis because in the condensed state of chromosomes, there is little or no RNA synthesis.

(c) The *ribosome* is the structure where various RNAs, enzymes, and other molecular species assemble the primary sequence of a protein. That is, amino acids are placed in order as specified by messenger RNA. Ribosomes are relatively nonspecific in that virtually any ribosome can be used in the translation of any mRNA. The structure and function of the ribosome will be described in greater detail in later chapters of the text.

(d) The *mitochondrion* (pl. *mitochondria*) is a membrane-bound structure located in the cytoplasm of eukaryotic cells. It is the site of oxidative phosphorylation and production of relatively large amounts of ATP, the energy currency of the cell, which drives many important metabolic processes in living systems.

(e) The *centriole* is a cytoplasmic structure involved (through the formation of spindle fibers) in the migration of chromosomes during mitosis and meiosis – primarily in animal cells.

(f) The *centromere* serves as an attachment point for sister chromatids (see F2.3, F2.4) and as a region where spindle fibers attach to chromosomes (kinetochore). The centromere divides during mitosis and meiosis II, thus aiding in the partitioning of chromosomal material to daughter cells. Failure of centromeres or spindle fibers to function properly may result in nondisjunction.

4. One of the most important concepts to be gained from this chapter is the relationship that exists among chromosomes in a single cell. Chromosomes that are homologous share many properties, including the following:

Overall length. Look carefully at F2.4 in this handbook to see that each cell, prior to anaphase I, contains two chromosomes, each with a homolog of approximately the same overall length.

Position of the centromere (metacentric, submetacentric, acrocentric, telocentric). Look carefully at F2.3 and again at F2.4, both in this handbook. Notice that if there is one metacentric chromosome, there will be another metacentric chromosome.

Banding patterns. Using various cytological techniques, bands can be visualized in chromosomes. In humans, homologous chromosomes of pair 1, for example, will have the same banding pattern. Although the overall length of chromosome pairs 16 and 17 appears to be the same, the banding patterns of these nonhomologous chromosomes will be different. (See Figure 2.4 in the textbook.)

Sister chromatids have identical banding patterns, as would be expected because sister chromatids are, with the exception of mutation or crossing over, identical copies of each other, generated by DNA replication. We would expect that homologous chromosomes would have banding patterns that are very similar (but not identical) because homologous chromosomes are genetically similar but not genetically identical.

Type and location of genes. A locus signifies the location of a gene along a chromosome (see F2.2 in this handbook, gene *A* or gene *B*). Thus, for each characteristic specified by a gene (such as blood type, eye color, or skin pigmentation), there are genes located along the chromosomes. The *order* of such loci is identical in homologous chromosomes, but the genes themselves may not be identical. F2.2 shows alternative forms of genes (alleles), *A* and *a*, on the metacentric chromosome pair. *A* and *a* are located at the same place and specify the same *characteristic* (seed color in peas, for example), but are slightly different manifestations of that trait (yellow vs. green, for example). Just as an individual may inherit allele *A* from the father and allele *a* from the mother for a given gene, each zygote inherits one homolog of each chromosome pair from the father and one homolog of each pair from the mother.

Diploidy is a term often used in conjunction with the symbol 2*n*. It means that there are two complete sets of chromosomes in the genome present in the cell. In humans, the diploid chromosome number is 46, whereas in *Drosophila melanogaster*, it is 8. The text lists the *haploid* chromosome number for a variety of species.

Haploidy refers to the fact that each haploid cell contains *one complete set of chromosomes* characterized for the species. The haploid chromosome number is one-half the diploid number and is usually symbolized as *n*.

Compare the nuclear contents of a spermatid with that of a primary spermatocyte at the end of prophase I (see text Figure 2.11). Note that each spermatid contains one member of each of the original chromosome pairs. The change from diploid (2*n*) to haploid (*n*) occurs when tetrads become dyads during meiosis I. Referring to the number of human chromosomes, the primary spermatocyte (2*n* = 46) becomes two secondary spermatocytes, each with *n* = 23.

5. As you examine the criteria for *homology* in Problem 4, you can see that overall length and centromere position are but two factors required for homology. Most important, genetic content in nonhomologous chromosomes is expected to be quite different. Other factors, including banding pattern, would also be expected to vary among nonhomologous chromosomes.

6. Because a major section of Chapter 2 deals with mitosis, it would be best to deal with this question by reviewing the appropriate section in the text and examining the corresponding figures. Understanding mitosis and all of the related terms is essential for an understanding of genetics.

7. Refer to text Figure 2.3. A chromosome with the centromere located in the middle is called metacentric. When the centromere is between the middle and the end of the chromosome, it is called submetacentric. In acrocentric chromosomes, the centromere is close to the end, and chromosomes with the centromere at the end are called telocentric. The following figure shows the different anaphase shapes of chromosomes as each moves toward a pole to the left: metacentric (a), submetacentric (b), acrocentric (c), and telocentric (d).

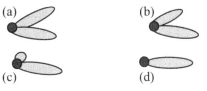

8. The mechanism of cytokinesis differs between these two cell types. In animal cells, constriction of the cell membrane produces a cell furrow and ultimately divides the parent cell. In plant cells, a new cell wall must be constructed around the plasma membrane. To do this, a cell plate is laid down during telophase and becomes the middle lamella. Next, the primary and secondary layers of the cell wall are deposited and two daughter cells result.

9. Carefully read the section on mitosis and cell division in the text. Major divisions of the cell cycle include interphase and mitosis. Interphase is composed of three phases: G1, S, and G2. (Some cells have a temporary or permanent G0 phase between G1 and S.) During the S phase, chromosomal DNA doubles. Karyokinesis involves nuclear division, whereas cytokinesis involves division of the cytoplasm. Refer to F2.1 for information pertaining to interphase. Refer to the text figures for a diagram of mitosis. Notice that in contrast to meiosis, there is no pairing of homologous chromosomes in mitosis and the chromosome number does not change.

10. (a) *Synapsis* is the point-by-point pairing of homologous chromosomes during prophase of meiosis I.

(b) *Bivalents* are those structures formed by the synapsis of homologous chromosomes: There are two replicated chromosomes (thus four chromatids) that make up a bivalent. If an organism has a diploid chromosome number of 46, then there will be 23 bivalents in meiosis I.

(c) *Chiasmata* is the plural form of *chiasma* and refers to the structure, when viewed microscopically, representing areas of crossing over between chromatids

(d) *Crossing over* is the exchange of genetic material between chromatids and a form of recombination. It is a method of providing genetic variation through the breaking and rejoining of chromatids.

(e) *Sister chromatids* are "post–S phase" structures of replicated chromosomes (see F2.1 and F2.2 in this handbook). Sister chromatids are genetically identical (except where mutations or crossovers have occurred) and are originally attached at the centromere. They separate from each other during anaphase of mitosis and anaphase II of meiosis.

(f) *Tetrads* are synapsed homologous chromosomes and thereby composed of four chromatids. There are as many tetrads as the haploid chromosome number.

(g) *Dyads* are replicated chromosomes, composed of two sister chromatids that are joined at a centromere. Each tetrad is made of two dyads that separate from each other during anaphase I of meiosis.

(h) *Monads*, or daughter chromosomes, result when the centromeres of dyads divide at anaphase II of meiosis.

11. Sister chromatids are the result of replication of a specific chromosome and are maintained together via the kinetochore and the cohesin protein complex. Before the process of meiosis, sister chromatids are genetically identical, except where mutations may have occurred during DNA replication. Nonsister chromatids are the replicated copies of another chromosome, although the term is generally used to refer to the duplicates of the other chromosome in a homologous pair. Nonsister chromatids will be genetically dissimilar if comparing nonhomologous chromosomes, but genetically similar (same gene order but with possible differences at the sequence level) if comparing homologous chromosomes. If crossing over and genetic recombination occur, then chromatids attached to the same centromere may no longer be identical.

12. During meiosis I, the chromosome number is reduced to haploid complements. This is achieved by pairing and synapsis of homologous chromosomes and their subsequent separation in anaphase I. During mitosis, chromosome number and content are maintained. If homologous chromosomes paired, it would be mechanically difficult to separate all sister chromatids to produce two identical daughter nuclei. However, by having chromosomes unpaired at metaphase of mitosis, only centromere division is required for daughter cells to eventually receive identical chromosomal complements.

13. Examine appropriate figures in the text. Notice that major differences include the sex in which each occurs and that the distribution of cytoplasm is unequal in oogenesis but considered to be equal in the products of spermatogenesis. Chromosomal behavior is the same in spermatogenesis and oogenesis except that the positioning of the metaphase plate in oogenesis is "off-center," thereby producing first and second polar bodies by unequal cytoplasmic division.

Via meiosis, each primary spermatocyte produces four spermatids, whereas each primary oocyte produces one ootid. Because early development occurs in the absence of outside nutrients, it is likely that the unequal distribution of cytoplasm in oogenesis evolved to provide sufficient information and nutrients to support development until the transcriptional activities of the zygotic nucleus begin to provide products. Polar bodies probably represent nonfunctional by-products of such evolution.

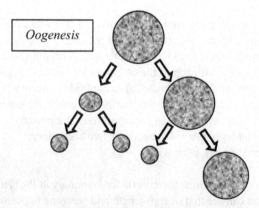

14. First, through independent assortment of chromosomes at anaphase I of meiosis, daughter cells (secondary spermatocytes and secondary oocytes) may contain different sets of maternally and paternally derived chromosomes and therefore different versions of genes (segregation of alleles). Examine the diagram that follows. Notice that there are several ways in which the maternally and paternally derived chromosomes may align. Second, crossing over, which happens at a much higher frequency in meiotic cells as compared to mitotic cells, allows maternally and paternally derived chromosomes to exchange segments, thereby increasing the likelihood that daughter cells (that is, secondary spermatocytes and secondary oocytes) are genetically unique.

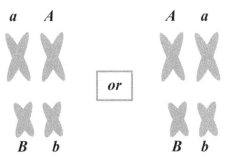

By contrast, daughter cells resulting from mitosis are usually genetically identical because there is no mechanism for independent assortment of chromosomes and traditional crossing over does not occur.

15. This question specifically tests your understanding of mitosis and meiosis and the behavior of chromosomes during the distinct anaphases. For this question, you must first visualize the alignment of the three homologous chromosome pairs C1/C2, M1/M2, and S1/S2 in mitosis, where there is no pairing or synapsis.

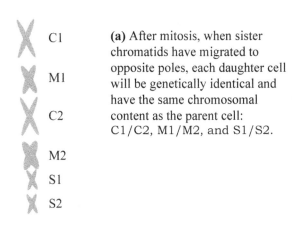

(a) After mitosis, when sister chromatids have migrated to opposite poles, each daughter cell will be genetically identical and have the same chromosomal content as the parent cell: C1/C2, M1/M2, and S1/S2.

(b) The first meiotic metaphase will have the following general configuration.

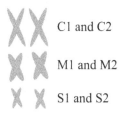

C1 and C2

M1 and M2

S1 and S2

(c) For the haploid products of the cell in part **(b)**, there are eight (2^n, where n = number of homolog pairs) different combinations of alignments possible because the members of each pair have two possible orientations.

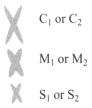

C_1 or C_2

M_1 or M_2

S_1 or S_2

16. If there are eight (2^3) combinations possible in part **(c)** in the previous problem, there would be 16 combinations (2^4) with the addition of another chromosome pair.

17. As you first read this question, think about an animal with $n = 6$; therefore, in the diploid parent cell, there will be six tetrads. All of these tetrads pass normally through meiosis I, which means six dyads go to each daughter cell. If one dyad undergoes secondary nondisjunction, which occurs during the second meiotic division, this would result in five chromosomes in one daughter nucleus and seven in the other.

(a) The mature ovum should contain $n + 1$ chromosomes ($6 + 1 = 7$): five chromosomes from normal disjunction and two chromosomes from the nondisjunction of one of the dyads.

(b) The second polar body did not receive one of the six monads it would normally receive, so it should have five monads (which are individual chromosomes).

(c) When the normal sperm with its n chromosome number combines with an $n + 1$ ovum, it will produce a zygote with $2n + 1$, or 13, chromosomes. While there will be two pairs of five kinds of chromosomes, there will be three of one kind of chromosome This condition is termed *trisomy*.

18. One-half of each tetrad will have a maternal homolog, so the probability of a maternal homolog is 1/2. Since there are 10 tetrads, $p = (1/2)^{10}$ for a sperm with only maternal homologs.

19. 0.72 picograms; 0.36 picograms; and 0.72 picograms.

The DNA content of a diploid cell will be twice that of the haploid cell. A diploid cell that has undergone DNA replication will have twice the DNA content as it did before replication.

20. In multicellular plants, the diploid sporophyte stage predominates. Meiosis results in the formation of the haploid male and female gametophyte stage, producing pollen and ovules respectively. Following fertilization, the sporophyte is formed.

21. The chromatin fiber is typically viewed as the 30 nm DNA plus nucleosome structure, whereas mitotic chromosomes are the highly compacted, densely folded form of chromatin. The transition from chromatin to individual chromosomes occurs at the beginning of mitosis (or meiosis). During this time, chromatin fibers fold up and condense into the typical mitotic chromosome. The folded-fiber model depicts this transition.

22. The folded-fiber model depicts each chromatid as a single fiber that becomes wound like a skein of yarn. Each fiber consists of DNA and protein. A coiling process occurs during the transition from interphase chromatin to more condensed chromosomes during prophase of mitosis or meiosis. Such condensation leads to a 5000-fold contraction in the length of the DNA within each chromatid. This eventually leads to the typically shortened and "fattened" metaphase chromosome.

23. They are likely to be homologous chromosomes and should contain similar (but not identical) genetic information. As homologous chromosomes, they would display the following characteristics. Their centromeres would most likely be in the same position relative to chromosome arm lengths (as noted), and any physical characteristics such as secondary constrictions or bands would be similar. Additionally, they would have a similar sequence of nitrogenous bases.

24. 50, 50, 50, 100, 200

25. Duplicated chromosomes A^m, A^p, B^m, B^p, C^m, and C^p will align individually at metaphase. Centromeres will divide and sister chromatids (now daughter chromosomes) will be pulled to opposite poles at anaphase. Both daughter cells will receive a copy of each of the six chromosomes.

26. At the end of prophase I, maternal and paternal copies of each homologous chromosome (A^m and A^p, B^m and B^p, and C^m and C^p) will be have completed synapsis and begun to pull apart. Side-by-side alignment of A^m with A^p, B^m with B^p, and C^m with C^p will occur in various arrangements at metaphase I. Eight possible combinations of products will occur at the completion of anaphase I: A^m, B^p, C^m, for example (each with sister chromatids). In other words, after meiosis I, the two product cells would be as follows: A^m or A^p, B^m or B^p, C^m or C^p.

27. As long as you have accounted for eight possible combinations in the previous problem, there would be no new ones added in this problem.

28. Eight $(2 \times 2 \times 2)$ combinations are possible.

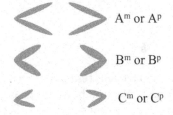

A^m or A^p

B^m or B^p

C^m or C^p

29. See the products of nondisjunction of chromosome C at the end of meiosis I as follows:

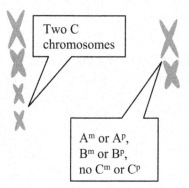

Two C chromosomes

A^m or A^p, B^m or B^p, no C^m or C^p

You are told that the C chromosomes separate as dyads instead of monads during meiosis II. There are two possible outcomes for late anaphase/early telophase, shown below. In the first (left-hand figure), the C chromosomes move as dyads into one of the two daughter nuclei (a second nondisjunction event). As a result, at the end of meiosis, one cell would contain single monads for the A and B chromosomes and two monads of the C chromosome. The other two cells would contain only the monads for chromosomes A and B, with no C chromosome. In the second possibility (right-hand figure), the C chromosome dyads separate from one another, resulting in two cells each containing monads for the A and B chromosomes and two monads of the C chromosome. The other two cells are as described previously.

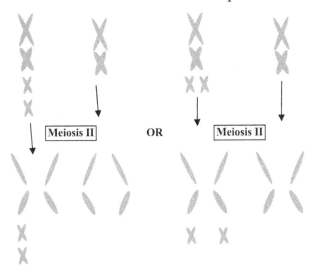

Under the second possibility depicted in problem 29, one would expect the following zygotes after fertilization:

zygotes 1–2:   two copies of chromosome A
two copies of chromosome B
three copies of chromosome C

zygotes 3–4:   two copies of chromosome A
two copies of chromosome B
one copy of chromosome C

None of the zygotes will be diploid.

30. Continuing with the gamete possibilities described in problem 29—nondisjunction of the C chromosome at meiosis I and again, nondisjunction of the same chromosome at meiosis II, you will end up, after fertilization by a normal gamete, with the following combinations:

zygote 1:   two copies of chromosome A
two copies of chromosome B
five copies of chromosome C

zygotes 2–4:   two copies of chromosome A
two copies of chromosome B
one copy of chromosome C

Chapter 3: Mendelian Genetics

<u>Concept Areas</u>	<u>Corresponding Problems</u>
Mendel's Postulates	1, 2, 5, 6, 9, 10, 11, 15, 16, 21, 22, 23, 24
Monohybrid Crosses	3, 4, 9, 11, 15, 16, 24
Homology	2, 10, 11
Probability	4, 18, 19, 20, 23
Dihybrid Crosses	7, 8, 9, 12, 13, 14
Trihybrid and Other Multifactor Crosses	13, 18, 19, 20, 23
Independent Assortment	7, 8, 9, 10, 12, 13, 14, 18, 19, 20, 23
Chi-Square Analysis	1, 15, 16, 17, 24
Pedigree Analysis	1, 21, 22

Structures and Processes Checklist—Significant items that deserve special attention are identified with a "*".

(Check topic when mastered–provide examples where appropriate–understand the context of each entry)

- **Overview**
  - Gregor Johann Mendel, 1866
  - *Pisum sativum*
  - discrete units of inheritance*
  - transmission genetics
- **Mendel's Experimental Approach**
  - patterns of inheritance*
  - artificial hybridization
  - contrasting pairs
  - traits
- **Transmission of One Trait**
  - monohybrid cross*
  - selfing
  - P_1, or parental generation
  - F_1, or first filial generation
  - F_2, or second filial generation

- 3:1 ratio
- reciprocal cross
- Mendel's postulates
- unit factor
- pairs
- dominance/recessiveness
- segregation
- modern terminology*
- phenotype*
- genes*
- alleles*
- genotype*
- homozygous*, homozygote
- heterozygous*, heterozygote
- Punnett square*
- testcross*

- **Mendel's Dihybrid Cross***
  - dihybrid, or two-factor, cross*
  - product law*
  - simultaneous independent events
  - Mendel's fourth postulate
  - independent assortment*
  - Mendel's 9:3:3:1 dihybrid ratio*
- **Inheritance of Multiple Traits**
  - trihybrid, or three-factor, cross
  - forked-line method or branch diagram
  - 27:9:9:9:3:3:3:1 ratio
- **Rediscovery of Mendel's Work***
  - Flemming, 1879
  - de Vries, Correns, Tschermak
  - Sutton, Boveri
  - chromosome theory of inheritance*
  - correlations*
  - diploid number $(2n)$*
  - maternal parent
  - paternal parent
  - Mendel's unit factors*
  - homologous chromosome pairs*
  - locus (pl. loci)
- **Independent Assortment***
  - extensive genetic variation
  - 2^n*
- **Laws of Probability***
  - product law*
  - sum law*

- large sample size
- **Chi-Square Analysis***
  - chance deviation
  - null hypothesis (H_0)*
  - chi-square (χ^2) analysis
  - $\chi^2 = \Sigma \dfrac{(o-e)^2}{e}$
  - degrees of freedom (df)*
  - probability value (p)*
  - interpreting probability values*
  - standard of $p = 0.05$
  - failure to reject the null hypothesis $(p > 0.05)$
  - rejection of the null hypothesis $(p < 0.05)$
  - reassess assumptions
  - significant difference*
- **Patterns of Inheritance in Humans**
  - pedigree*
  - pedigree conventions*
  - consanguineous*
  - sibs, siblings
  - sibship line
  - Arabic numerals (birth order)
  - Roman numerals (generations)
  - shaded (expressed)* unshaded (not expressed)*
  - diagonal line (deceased)
  - monozygotic, or identical, twins*
  - dizygotic, or fraternal, twins*

- proband (p)
- pedigree analysis
- albinism (recessive)
- Huntington disease (dominant)
- familial hypercholesterolemia
- LDL

- **Molecular Basis of a Disorder**
  - Tay–Sachs disease
  - hexosaminidase A (Hex-A)
  - ganglioside GM2

F3.1 Illustration of the union of maternal and paternal gametes, each carrying a copy of the specific gene, to give a gene pair to the resulting zygote. Mendelian "unit factors" occur in pairs in diploid organisms this way. Dominant alleles are often given the uppercase letter for their symbol, whereas the lowercase letter is often used to symbolize the recessive allele.

a) Note that each parent contributes one chromosome of each homologous chromosome pair and, thus, one gene of each gene pair.

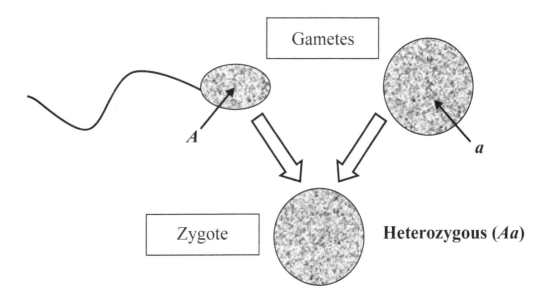

b) Arrangement of genes on homologous chromosomes; viewed as metaphase chromosomes

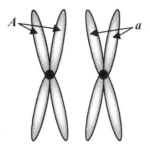

F3.2 Critical symbolism associated with genes and chromosomes. A locus (pl. loci) is the location of a gene on a chromosome. Pictured here, two gene loci (one for gene *A* and another for gene *B*) are shown on nonhomologous metaphase chromosomes. Note that with two different gene pairs, two different characteristics may be involved, such as seed shape (*A* and *a*) and seed color (*B* and *b*).

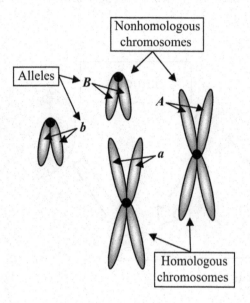

F3.3 One of the most important concepts for this section is illustrated in this figure. Two genes (*W* and *B*) are presented, each representing a different characteristic: seed shape (alleles *W* and *w*) and seed color (alleles *B* and *b*). Different genes may influence completely different characteristics (as indicated here) or the same characteristic (described in Chapter 4).

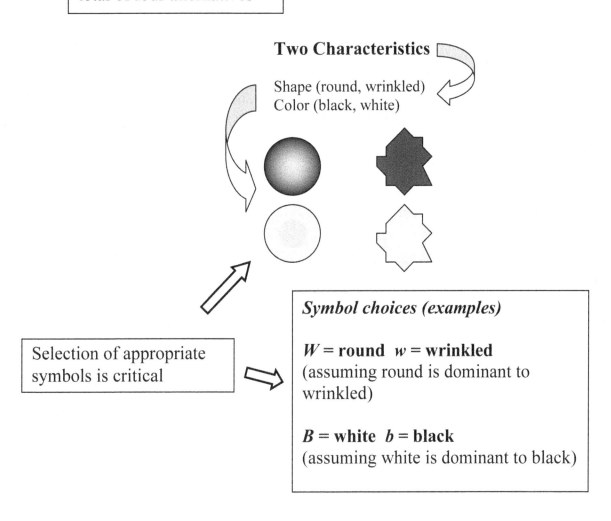

Two characteristics but a total of four alternatives

Two Characteristics

Shape (round, wrinkled)
Color (black, white)

Selection of appropriate symbols is critical

Symbol choices (examples)

W = **round** *w* = **wrinkled**
(assuming round is dominant to wrinkled)

B = **white** *b* = **black**
(assuming white is dominant to black)

Chapter 3 *Mendelian Genetics*

Answers to Now Solve This

3.1 First, read the entire question and see that you are to determine the pattern of inheritance for one characteristic, *pattern*, with two alternatives, checkered vs. plain. We should consider this a monohybrid scenario unless complications arise. Assignment of symbols:

P = checkered; p = plain

Checkered is tentatively assigned the dominant function because, in a casual examination of the data, we see that in crosses between checkered and plain individuals, checkered types are present in both F_1 and F_2 generations whereas plain types disappear in the F_1 generation [see cross (b)] and reappear in the F_2 generation [see cross (f)].

Cross (a):

$PP \times PP$ or $PP \times Pp$

To distinguish between these possibilities, look at crosses (d) and (g). In cross (d), a test cross, only checkered F_2 progeny are produced in multiple crosses between the checkered offspring of cross (a) and plain offspring of cross (c). Furthermore, cross (g) also shows only checkered progeny when multiple checkered offspring of cross (a) are mated to heterozygous checkered offspring of cross (b) [see below]. Together, these data argue strongly that there are no heterozygotes in the progeny of cross (a), and that the original cross must have been $PP \times PP$.

[Note: it is still possible, but less probable, that the second parent of cross (a) was heterozygous, and that heterozygous F_1 offspring were undetected because not all the offspring were tested in further crosses.]

Cross (b):

$PP \times pp$

This assignment seems reasonable because among 38 offspring, no plain types are produced. In addition, we would expect all the F_1 progeny to be heterozygous, and if crossed to plain, as in cross (e), to produce approximately half checkered and half plain offspring. In cross (f), we would expect such heterozygotes to produce a 3:1 ratio, which is observed.

Cross (c):

$pp \times pp$

Because all of the offspring from this cross are plain, there is no doubt that the genotype of both parents is pp.

Genotypes of all individuals:

		Progeny	
	P₁ Cross	**Checkered**	**Plain**
(a)	$PP \times PP$	PP	
(b)	$PP \times pp$	Pp	
(c)	$pp \times pp$		pp
	F₁ x F₁ Cross	**Checkered**	**Plain**
(d)	$PP \times pp$	Pp	
(e)	$Pp \times pp$	Pp	pp
(f)	$Pp \times Pp$	PP, Pp	pp
(g)	$PP \times Pp$	PP, Pp	

3.2 Symbolism as before:

w = wrinkled seeds	g = green cotyledons
W = round seeds	G = yellow cotyledons

26

Examine each characteristic (seed shape vs. cotyledon color) separately.

(a) Notice a 3:1 ratio for seed shape; therefore, $Ww \times Ww$, and no green cotyledons; therefore, $GG \times GG$ or $GG \times Gg$. (Note: one parent must be GG while the other parent can be either GG or Gg). Putting the two characteristics together gives

   $WwGG \times WwGG$

       or

   $WwGG \times WwGg$

(b) There is a 1:1 ratio for seed shape (8/16 wrinkled and 8/16 round) and a 3:1 ratio for cotyledon color (12/16 yellow and 4/16 green). Therefore, the answer is

   $WwGg \times wwGg$

(c) $WwGg \times WwGg$ a standard dihybrid cross

(d) This is a typical 1:1:1:1 testcross ratio and signifies that one parent is doubly heterozygous, whereas the other is fully homozygous recessive. The answer is

   $WwGg \times wwgg$

3.3 (a) When examining the cross $AaBbCc \times AaBBCC$, expect there to be eight (2^n, where $n =$ number of heterozygous loci) different kinds of gametes from one parent ($AaBbCc$) and two different kinds from the other ($AaBBCC$). Therefore, there should be 16 different genotypes among the offspring (8×2). Using the forked-line method:

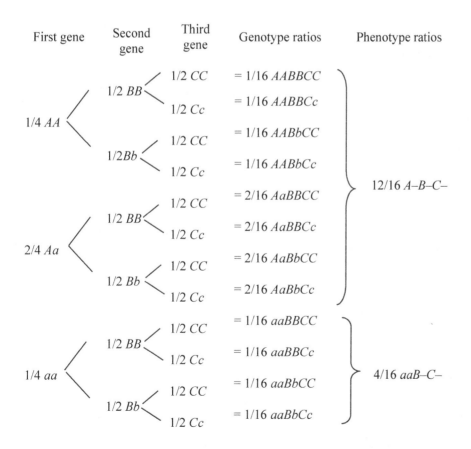

Notice that a dash (–) is used where, because of dominance, it makes no difference as to the dominant/recessive status of the second allele for that gene.

(b) There will be four kinds of gametes for the first parent (*AaBBCc*) and two kinds of gametes for the second parent (*aaBBCc*). Therefore, there should be eight different genotypes among the offspring (4 × 2).

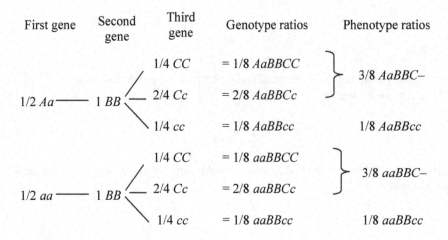

First gene	Second gene	Third gene	Genotype ratios	Phenotype ratios

1/2 *Aa* —— 1 *BB*
- 1/4 *CC* = 1/8 *AaBBCC* ⎫
- 2/4 *Cc* = 2/8 *AaBBCc* ⎬ 3/8 *AaBBC–*
- 1/4 *cc* = 1/8 *AaBBcc* 1/8 *AaBBcc*

1/2 *aa* —— 1 *BB*
- 1/4 *CC* = 1/8 *aaBBCC* ⎫
- 2/4 *Cc* = 2/8 *aaBBCc* ⎬ 3/8 *aaBBC–*
- 1/4 *cc* = 1/8 *aaBBcc* 1/8 *aaBBcc*

(c) There will be eight different kinds of gametes from each of the parents and therefore a 64-box Punnett square. Doing this problem by the forked-line method helps considerably.

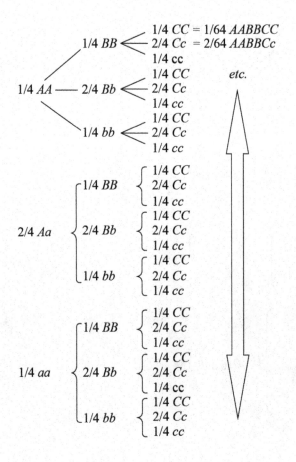

1/4 *AA* —— 2/4 *Bb*
- 1/4 *BB*
  - 1/4 *CC* = 1/64 *AABBCC*
  - 2/4 *Cc* = 2/64 *AABBCc*
  - 1/4 *cc*
- 2/4 *Bb*
  - 1/4 *CC*
  - 2/4 *Cc*
  - 1/4 *cc*
- 1/4 *bb*
  - 1/4 *CC*
  - 2/4 *Cc*
  - 1/4 *cc*

etc.

2/4 *Aa*
- 1/4 *BB*
  - 1/4 *CC*
  - 2/4 *Cc*
  - 1/4 *cc*
- 2/4 *Bb*
  - 1/4 *CC*
  - 2/4 *Cc*
  - 1/4 *cc*
- 1/4 *bb*
  - 1/4 *CC*
  - 2/4 *Cc*
  - 1/4 *cc*

1/4 *aa*
- 1/4 *BB*
  - 1/4 *CC*
  - 2/4 *Cc*
  - 1/4 *cc*
- 2/4 *Bb*
  - 1/4 *CC*
  - 2/4 *Cc*
  - 1/4 *cc*
- 1/4 *bb*
  - 1/4 *CC*
  - 2/4 *Cc*
  - 1/4 *cc*

Simply multiply through each component to arrive at the final genotypic frequencies.

For the phenotypic frequencies, set up the problem in the following manner:

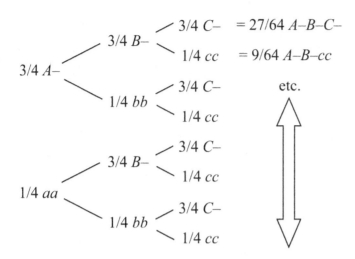

3.4 (a) Think of this problem as a dihybrid F_2 situation. Set up a table following the format of Table 3.1 of the text.:

Expected ratio	Observed (o)	Expected (e)	Deviation ($o - e = d$)	Deviation^2	d^2/e
9/16	315	9/16 × 556 =312.75	315 - 312.75 =2.25	$(2.25)^2 = 5.0625$	5.0625/312.75 = 0.016
3/16	108	3/16 × 556 =104.25	108 - 104.25 = 3.75	$(3.75)^2 = 14.0625$	14.0625/104.25 = 0.135
3/16	101	3/16 × 556 =104.25	101 − 104.25 = -3.25	$(-3.25)^2 = 10.5623$	10.5623/104.25 = 0.101
1/16	32	1/16 × 556 =34.75	32 - 34.75 = -2.75	$(-2.75)^2 = 7.5625$	7.5625/34.75 = 0.218
	Total = 556				$\chi^2 = 0.47$

Looking at the table in the text, you can see that this χ^2 value is associated with a probability greater than 0.90 for 3 degrees of freedom (because there are four classes in the χ^2 test). We fail to reject the null hypothesis and are confident that the observed values do not differ significantly from the expected values.

To deal with parts **(b)** and **(c)**, it is easier to see the observed values for the monohybrid ratios if the phenotypes are listed:

smooth, yellow	315
smooth, green	108
wrinkled, yellow	101
wrinkled, green	32

(b) For the smooth:wrinkled *monohybrid component*, the smooth types total 423 (315 + 108), whereas the wrinkled types total 133 (101 + 32).

Expected ratio	Observed (o)	Expected (e)	Deviation ($o - e = d$)	Deviation^2	d^2/e
3/4	423	417	6	36	0.086
1/4	133	139	-6	36	0.259
	Total = 556				$\chi^2 = 0.345$

The χ^2 value is 0.35; in examining the text for 1 degree of freedom (there are two classes), the *p* value is greater than 0.50 and less than 0.90. We fail to reject the null hypothesis and are confident that the observed values do not differ significantly from the expected values.

(c) For the yellow:green portion of the problem, there are 416 yellow plants (315 + 101) and 140 (108 + 32) green plants.

Expected ratio	Observed (o)	Expected (e)	Deviation ($o - e = d$)	Deviation^2	d^2/e
3/4	416	417	-1	1	0.0024
1/4	140	139	1	1	0.0072
	Total = 556				$\chi^2 = 0.01$

The χ^2 value is 0.01; in examining the text for 1 degree of freedom, the *p* value is greater than 0.90. We fail to reject the null hypothesis and are confident that the observed values do not differ significantly from the expected values.

3.5 The gene is inherited as an autosomal recessive. The key observation is that two normal individuals (II-3 and II-4) have produced a daughter (III-2) with myopia. Symbolism: *m* = myopic and *M* = normal vision

    I-1 (*mm*), I-2 (*Mm* or *MM*), I-3 (*Mm*), I-4 (*Mm*)

    II-1 (*Mm*), II-2 (*Mm*), II-3 (*Mm*), II-4 (*Mm*), II-5 (*mm*), II-6 (*MM* or *Mm*), II-7 (*MM* or *Mm*)

    III-1 (*MM* or *Mm*), III-2 (*mm*), III-3 (*MM* or *Mm*)

Chapter 3 Mendelian Genetics

Solutions to Problems and Discussion Questions

1. (a) By noting that traits passed unaltered from parental to subsequent generations, Mendel not only postulated the "unit" or "particulate" nature of hereditary elements, but he also described their behavior. Results of various crosses provided the basis for knowing that factors can remain hidden in some circumstances, thereby implying two participating elements, one dominating the other. Predictable ratios in crosses supported the hypothesis of two hereditary elements involved in the expression of a given trait.

(b) Typically, by conducting a testcross, one readily tests whether an organism is homozygous or heterozygous for the dominant trait.

(c) In general, a chi-square analysis is used to compare observed data with various genetic models.

(d) Pedigree analysis is often used to determine whether and how traits are inherited in humans. However, other methods are also used and are discussed in subsequent chapters.

2. Your essay should include the following:
(1) Factors occur in pairs. Given the diploid nature of many organisms, alleles on one chromosome often have an allele on a homologous chromosome.

(2) Some genes have dominant and recessive alleles. In many cases, one allele is capable of causing a "wild type" or common function in the presence of a mutant allele.

(3) Alleles segregate from each other during gamete formation. When homologous chromosomes separate from each other at anaphase I, alleles will go to opposite poles of the meiotic apparatus and are then destined to separate gametes.

(4) One gene pair separates independently from other gene pairs. Different gene pairs on nonhomologous chromosomes or, if far enough apart, on the same homologous pair of chromosomes will separate independently from each other during meiosis.

3. The first sentence of this question indicates that one characteristic (coat color) with two alternatives (black and white) is being described; therefore, a monohybrid scenario exists.

You can also deduce which allele, *black* or *white*, is dominant. The problem indicates that all of the offspring from a cross of black × white parents are black; therefore, black can be considered dominant. The second sentence of the problem

verifies that a monohybrid cross is involved because of the 3/4 black and 1/4 white distribution in the F_2 offspring.

Referring to appropriate text figures and knowing that genes occur in pairs in diploid organisms, one can write the genotypes and the phenotypes requested as follows:

P_1:			
Phenotypes:	black	×	white
Genotypes:	*WW*		*ww*
Gametes:	Ⓦ		ⓦ
F_1:	*Ww* (black)		

F_1 × F_1:			
Phenotypes:	black	×	black
Genotypes:	*Ww*		*Ww*
Gametes:	Ⓦ ⓦ	Ⓦ ⓦ	
	(combine as in the text)		

F_2:

Phenotypes:	black	black	black	white
Genotypes:	*WW*	*Ww*	*Ww*	*ww*

4. Start out with the following gene symbols:

A = without albinism,
a = with albinism.

Albinism is inherited as a recessive trait, so individuals without albinism will have a genotype of *AA* or *Aa*, whereas individuals with albinism will have a genotype of *aa*.

(a) The parents are both unaffected; therefore, they could be either *AA* or *Aa*. Because they produced a child with albinism, each parent must have provided an *a* allele to the child; thus, both parents must be heterozygous (*Aa*).

(b) The unaffected male could have either the *AA* or *Aa* genotype. The female must be *aa*. Because all of the children are unaffected, one would consider it more likely that the male is *AA* instead of *Aa*. However, it *is* possible for the male to be *Aa*. Under that circumstance, the likelihood of having six children, all unaffected, is ½ x ½ x ½ x ½ x ½ x ½ = 1/64.

32

5. Mendel's first three postulates are illustrated in this problem. Postulate 1: Unit factors (genes) occur in pairs—unaffected parents can be homozygous or heterozygous. Postulate 2: Alleles demonstrate dominance/recessive relationships—heterozygous individuals are unaffected because they possess one dominant allele. Postulate 3: Segregation of alleles - unit factors separate from each other during gamete formation.

6. *Pisum sativum* is easy to cultivate and is naturally self-fertilizing, but it can be crossbred. It has numerous visible features (for example, tall or short, red flowers or white flowers) that are consistent under a variety of environmental conditions yet are easily distinguishable. Seeds could be obtained from local merchants.

7. Two *characteristics* are being studied: seed shape and cotyledon color. Therefore, this is a dihybrid situation with *two gene pairs* involved. Two alternatives are possible for each of these two characteristics: *seed shape*, wrinkled vs. round; *cotyledon color*, green vs. yellow. The phenotype of the F₁ plants allows you to deduce that the allele for round seeds is dominant to that for wrinkled seeds and the allele for yellow cotyledons is dominant to that for green cotyledons.

> Symbolism:
>
> w = wrinkled seeds   g = green cotyledons
>
> W = round seeds   G = yellow cotyledons

P₁:

>   *WWGG*   ×   *wwgg*

Parents are considered to be homozygous for two reasons. First, in the introductory sentence, just after "Problems and Discussion Questions," there is the statement "members of the P₁ generation are homozygous, unless …" The second, more scientific, reason is that the only offspring are those with round seeds and yellow cotyledons.

Gametes produced: One member of each gene pair is "segregated" to each gamete.

        WWGG   *wwgg*

F₁: *WwGg*

F₁   ×   F₁:

>   *WwGg*   ×   *WwGg*

Gametes produced: Under conditions of independent assortment, four (2^n, where n = number of heterozygous gene pairs) different types of gametes will be produced by each parent.

Punnett square:

	WG	*Wg*	*wG*	*wg*
WG	*WWGG*	*WWGg*	*WwGG*	*WwGg*
Wg	*WWGg*	*WWgg*	*WwGg*	*Wwgg*
wG	*WwGG*	*WwGg*	*wwGG*	*wwGg*
wg	*WwGg*	*Wwgg*	*wwGg*	*wwgg*

Collecting the phenotypes according to the dominance scheme just presented gives the following:

9/16 *W–G–* round seeds, yellow cotyledons
3/16 *W–gg* round seeds, green cotyledons
3/16 *wwG–* wrinkled seeds, yellow cotyledons
1/16 *wwgg* wrinkled seeds, green cotyledons

Again, notice that a dash (–) is used where, because of dominance, it makes no difference as to the dominant/recessive status of the allele.

Forked-line method or branch diagram:

Seed shape	Cotyledon color	Phenotypes

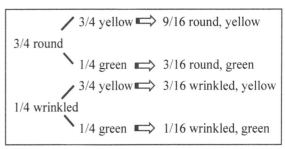

8. In a testcross, an individual that expresses the dominant phenotype but whose genotype is unknown is crossed to a fully homozygous recessive individual. Cross (d) of the Now Solve This problem 3.2, fits this description.

9. Problem 3 involves a monohybrid cross whereas Now Solve This problem 3.2 involves a dihybrid cross. While both problems demonstrate Mendel's first three postulates, only the latter demonstrates the fourth postulate—independent assortment, which states that segregation of one pair of genes is not influenced by segregation of any other gene pair.

10. (1) Mendel's paired unit factors correlate with pairs of genes, which are located on homologous chromosomes.
(2) Variants of genes (alleles) exhibit a dominant/recessive relationship (for example, round and wrinkled pea shape).
(3) The movement of homologous chromosomes to opposite poles of the spindle apparatus in anaphase I of meiosis correlates with the segregation of Mendel's paired unit factors during gamete formation.
(4) In meiosis, alignment and separation of one homologous chromosome pair does not affect that of another pair, just as Mendel's factors assorted independently of one another.

11. Homozygosity refers to a condition where both alleles of a gene pair are the same (for example, *AA* or *GG* or *hh*), whereas heterozygosity refers to the condition where members of a gene pair are different (for example, *Aa* or *Gg* or *Bb*). Homozygotes produce only one type of gamete, whereas heterozygotes will produce 2^n types of gametes, where n = number of heterozygous gene pairs (assuming independent assortment).

12. Two characteristics are presented here: body color and wing length. First, assign meaningful gene symbols.

Body color	*Wing length*
E = gray body color	*V* = long wings
e = ebony body color	*v* = vestigial wings

(a) P₁:

EEVV × *eevv*

F₁: *EeVv* (gray, long)

F₂: This will be the result of a Punnett square with 16 boxes, as in the text.

Phenotypes	*Ratio*	*Genotypes*	*Ratio*
gray, long	9/16	*EEVV*	1/16
		EEVv	2/16
		EeVV	2/16
		EeVv	4/16
gray, vestigial	3/16	*EEvv*	1/16
		Eevv	2/16
ebony, long	3/16	*eeVV*	1/16
		eeVv	2/16
ebony, vestigial	1/16	*eevv*	1/16

(b) P₁:

EEvv × *eeVV*

F₁: It is important to see that the results from this cross will be exactly the same as those in part **(a)**. The only difference is that the recessive alleles are coming from both parents rather than from one parent only as in **(a)**. The F₂ ratio will be the same as in **(a)** also. When you have genes on the autosomes (not X-linked), independent assortment, complete dominance, and no gene interaction (see later) in a cross involving double heterozygotes, the offspring ratio will be 9:3:3:1.

(c) P₁:

EEVV × *EEvv*

F₁: *EEVv* (gray, long)

F₂: Notice that all of the offspring will have gray bodies, and you will get a 3:1 ratio of long to vestigial wings. You should see this before you even begin working through the problem. Even though this cross involves two gene pairs, it will give a monohybrid type of ratio because one of the gene pairs is homozygous (body color) and one gene pair is heterozygous (wing length).

Phenotypes	*Ratio*	*Genotypes*	*Ratio*
gray, long	3/4	*EEVV*	1/4
		EEVv	2/4
gray, vestigial	1/4	*EEvv*	1/4

NOTE: After working through this problem, it is important that you try to work similar problems without constructing the time-consuming Punnett squares, especially if each problem asks for phenotypic rather than genotypic ratios.

13. The general formula for determining the number of kinds of gametes produced by an organism is 2^n, where n = number of *heterozygous* gene pairs.

(a) 4: *AB, Ab, aB, ab*

(b) 2: *AB, aB*

(c) 8: *ABC, ABc, AbC, Abc, aBC, aBc, abC, abc*

(d) 2: *ABc, aBc*

(e) 4: *ABc, Abc, aBc, abc*

(f) $2^5 = 32$

ABCDE	*aBCDE*
ABCDe	*aBCDe*
ABCdE	*aBCdE*
ABCde	*aBCde*
ABcDE	*aBcDE*
ABcDe	*aBcDe*
ABcdE	*aBcdE*
ABcde	*aBcde*
AbCDE	*abCDE*
AbCDe	*abCDe*
AbCdE	*abCdE*
AbCde	*abCde*
AbcDE	*abcDE*
AbcDe	*abcDe*
AbcdE	*abcdE*
Abcde	*abcde*

Notice that there is a pattern that can be used to write these gametes so that fewer errors will occur.

14. Two characteristics are being considered: seed color (yellow, green) and seed shape (round, wrinkled). At this point, you should be able to do this problem without writing down each of the steps. The F_1 can be considered to be a double heterozygote (with round and yellow being dominant). See the cross this way:

Symbols:

Seed shape	Seed color
W = round	*G* = yellow
w = wrinkled	*g* = green

P$_1$:   *WWgg* × *wwGG*

F$_1$:   *WwGg*

Testcross: *WwGg* × *wwgg*

Offspring will occur in a typical 1:1:1:1 ratio as

1/4 *WwGg* (round, yellow)

1/4 *Wwgg* (round, green)

1/4 *wwGg* (wrinkled, yellow)

1/4 *wwgg* (wrinkled, green)

Again, at this point, it would be very helpful if you could do such simple problems by inspection.

15. Because these are F$_2$ results from monohybrid crosses, a 3:1 ratio is expected for each. By referring to the text, one can set up the analysis easily.

(a)

Expected ratio	Observed (o)	Expected (e)
3/4	882	885.75
1/4	299	295.25

Expected values are derived by multiplying the expected ratio by the total number of organisms.

$$\chi^2 = \Sigma(o-e)^2/e = 0.064$$

In looking in the χ^2 table with 1 degree of freedom (because there were two classes, therefore, $n-1$ or 1 degree of freedom), we find a probability (p) value between 0.9 and 0.5.

We fail to reject the null hypothesis and say that there is a "good fit" between the observed and expected values. Notice that as the deviations between the observed and expected values increase, the value of χ^2 increases. So the higher the χ^2 value, the more likely it is that the null hypothesis will be rejected.

(b)

Expected ratio	Observed (o)	Expected (e)
3/4	705	696.75
1/4	224	232.25

$$\chi^2 = 0.39$$

The p value in the table for 1 degree of freedom is still between 0.9 and 0.5; however, because the χ^2

value is larger for **(b)**, we should say that the deviations from expectation are greater.

The deviation in each case can be attributed to chance.

16. It would be best to set up two tables based on the two hypotheses:

(a) Hypothesis: the data fit a 3:1 ratio.

Expected ratio	Observed (o)	Expected (e)
3/4	250	300
1/4	150	100

(b) Hypothesis: the data fit a 1:1 ratio.

Expected ratio	Observed (o)	Expected (e)
1/2	250	200
1/2	150	200

For the test of a 3:1 ratio, the χ^2 value is 33.3 with an associated *p* value of less than 0.01 for 1 degree of freedom. For the test of a 1:1 ratio, the χ^2 value is 25.0, again with an associated *p* value of less than 0.01 for 1 degree of freedom. Based on these probability values, both null hypotheses should be rejected.

17. Use of the $p = 0.10$ as the critical value for rejecting or failing to reject the null hypothesis instead of $p = 0.05$ would be a <u>more stringent</u> condition because it would allow more null hypotheses to be rejected. As the differences between observed and expected values increase, the χ^2 values also increase, so the higher the χ^2 value, the more likely the null hypothesis will be rejected. As the critical *p* value is increased, it takes a smaller χ^2 value (less difference between the expected and observed values) to cause rejection of the null hypothesis.

18. Given the cross $AaBbCC \times AABbCc$, we can apply the product rule, which states that when two or more events occur independently but simultaneously, their combined probability is equal to the product of their individual probabilities.

The probability of getting AA from

$Aa \quad \times \quad AA \quad$ is 1/2.

The probability of getting Bb from

$Bb \quad \times \quad Bb \quad$ is 1/2.

The probability of getting Cc from

$CC \quad \times \quad Cc \quad$ is 1/2.

The *overall* probability, then, is

$1/2 \quad \times \quad 1/2 \quad \times \quad 1/2 = 1/8.$

19. The probability of getting $aabbcc$ from the $AaBbCC \times AABbCc$ mating is zero because of homozygosity for AA in one parent and CC in the other.

20. All of the offspring will show the dominant A and C phenotypes and 3/4 will show the B phenotype. The probability of an offspring showing all three dominant traits would be the product of the probabilities at each locus:
$1 \times 3/4 \times 1 = 3/4$.

21. Although many different inheritance patterns will be described later in the text (codominance, incomplete dominance, sex-linked inheritance, etc.), the range of solutions to this question is limited to the concepts developed in the first three chapters, namely, dominance or recessiveness.

If an allele is dominant, it tends to be present in each generation, and will not be passed to offspring unless at least one of the parents expresses the allele. On the other hand, alleles that are recessive can skip generations and exist in a carrier state in parents. For example, in the pedigree, individuals II-4 and II-5 produce a female child (III-4) with the affected phenotype. On these criteria alone, the allele must be viewed as being autosomal recessive. (We will consider the pattern for X-linked recessive alleles in a later chapter.)

When providing genotypes for each individual, consider that if the box or circle is shaded, the *aa* genotype is to be assigned; a recessive allele must have come from each parent.

I-1 (*Aa*), I-2 (*aa*), I-3 (*Aa*), I-4 (*Aa*)

II-1 (*aa*), II-2 (*Aa*), II-3 (*aa*), II-4 (*Aa*), II-5 (*Aa*), II-6 (*aa*), II-7 (*AA* or *Aa*), II-8 (*AA* or *Aa*)

III-1 (*AA* or *Aa*), III-2 (*AA* or *Aa*), III-3 (*AA* or *Aa*), III-4 (*aa*), III-5 (*AA* or *Aa*; more likely *AA*), III-6 (*aa*)

IV-1 through IV-7 (all *Aa*)

22. (a) There are two possibilities. The trait could be dominant, in which case I-1 is heterozygous, as are II-2 and II-3, and the remaining individuals are homozygous recessive. Alternatively, the trait is recessive, I-1 is homozygous, and I-2 is heterozygous. Under the condition of recessiveness, both II-1 and II-4 would be heterozygous and II-2 and II-3 homozygous.

(b) Recessive: parents *Aa, Aa*

(c) Recessive: parents *Aa, Aa*

23. **(a)** First consider that each parent is homozygous (true-breeding in the question), and because in the F_1 only round, axial, violet, and full phenotypes were expressed, they must each be dominant. Because all genes are on nonhomologous chromosomes, independent assortment will occur.

(b) Round, axial, violet, and full would be the most frequent phenotypes:

$$3/4 \quad \times \quad 3/4 \quad \times \quad 3/4 \quad \times \quad 3/4 \quad = (3/4)^4$$

(c) Wrinkled, terminal, white, and constricted would be the least frequent phenotypes:

$$1/4 \quad \times \quad 1/4 \quad \times \quad 1/4 \quad \times \quad 1/4 \quad = (1/4)^4$$

(d) This question is asking for the probability of the round, terminal, violet, constricted phenotype OR the wrinkled, axial, white, full phenotype. Calculate the probability of each phenotype and apply the sum rule for the final probability of having *either* phenotype.

$(3/4 \times 1/4 \times 3/4 \times 1/4) + (1/4 \times 3/4 \times 1/4 \times 3/4) =$

$9/256 + 9/256 = 18/256 = 9/128$

(e) Calculate the number of different phenotypes in the offspring as for previous problems (for example,

see Now Solve This 3.3). There would be 16 different phenotypes in the testcross offspring.

24. **(a)** First, consider that the data represent a 3:1 ratio based on the information given in the problem: $Ss \times Ss$. Compute the expected quantities for each class by multiplying the totals by 3/4 and 1/4.

Set I expected numbers:

Tall = 26.25
Short = 8.75

Set II expected numbers:

Tall = 262.5
Short = 87.5

For set I, the χ^2 value would be

$(30 - 26.25)^2/26.25 + (5 - 8.75)^2/8.75$

= 2.14, with p being between 0.2 and 0.05.

We fail to reject the null hypothesis of no significant difference between the expected and observed values. For set II, the χ^2 value would be 21.43 and $p < 0.001$. A significant difference between the observed and expected values is found, so the null hypothesis is rejected.

(b) Clearly, with an increase in sample size, a different conclusion is reached. In fact, most statisticians recommend that the expected values in each class should not be less than 10. In most cases, more confidence is gained as the sample size increases; however, depending on the organism or experiment, there may be practical limits on sample size.

Chapter 4: Modification of Mendelian Ratios

Concept Areas	Corresponding Problems
Incomplete Dominance, Codominance	1, 3, 4, 6, 7, 11, 24, 26
Multiple Alleles	2, 4, 11, 23, 26
Lethal Alleles	1, 2, 5, 28
Gene Interaction	1, 8, 9, 16, 17, 18, 19, 33
Epistasis	1, 8, 9, 18, 19, 20, 22, 25, 32
Complementation	23
X-Linkage	1, 10, 11, 13, 14, 15, 16, 21, 27, 29, 34
Sex-Limited, Sex-Influenced	1, 12
Extranuclear Inheritance	1, 29, 30, 31

Structures and Processes Checklist—Significant items that deserve special attention are identified with a "*".

(Check topic when mastered–provide examples where appropriate–understand the context of each entry)

- **Overview**
  - complex modes of inheritance*
  - gene interaction
  - X-linkage
  - modification of Mendelian ratios
- **Alleles Alter Phenotypes**
  - wild-type allele*
  - mutant allele
  - loss-of-function mutation*
  - null allele*
  - gain-of-function mutation*
  - neutral mutation*
- **Symbols for Alleles***
  - italics
  - uppercase = dominant; lowercase = recessive (e.g., *D/d*)

- superscript + (e.g., e^+)
- slash – same locus on two homologs
- + symbol
- no dominance (e.g., R^1 and R^2 or L^M and L^N)
- **Neither Allele is Dominant***
  - incomplete, or partial, dominance*
  - 1:2:1, F_2 generation
  - Tay–Sachs disease
  - hexosaminidase A
- **Both Alleles Influence a Heterozygote**
  - joint expression of both alleles
  - codominance*
  - MN blood group
  - 1:2:1

- **Multiple Alleles of a Gene***
  - multiple alleles
  - studied only in populations*
  - ABO blood groups*
  - I^A, I^B, i
  - isoagglutinogen
  - H substance
  - Bombay phenotype
  - *fucosyl transferase* (*FUT1*) gene
  - *white* locus in *Drosophila*
  - allelic series

- **Lethal Alleles***
  - recessive lethal allele*
  - 2:1, surviving F_2 generation*
  - dominant lethal allele*
  - Huntington disease

- **Modified 9:3:3:1 Ratios***
  - combining two modes of inheritance*

- **Phenotypes Affected by More Than One Gene***
  - gene interaction*
  - epigenesis
  - hereditary deafness
  - heterogeneous trait
  - epistasis*
  - single trait followed
  - ratio expressed in 16 parts
  - recessive epistasis*
  - 9:3:4*

- dominant epistasis*
- 12:3:1*
- complementary gene interaction*
- 9:7*
- novel phenotypes*
- 9:6:1
- other modified dihybrid ratios
- 13:3
- 10:3:3
- 15:1
- 6:3:3:4

- **Complementation**
  - complementation analysis*
  - same gene or two different genes?
  - recessive mutations
  - complementation group

- **Multiple Effects of Single Gene***
  - pleiotropy*
  - Marfan syndrome
  - porphyria variegata

- **Genes on the X Chromosome**
  - X-linkage*
  - *white* eye-color mutation in *Drosophila*
  - different results for reciprocal crosses*
  - hemizygous*
  - crisscross pattern of inheritance*
  - chromosome theory of inheritance*
  - color blindness

Chapter 4 Modification of Mendelian Ratios

- **Gender Influences Phenotype**
  - genes not on X chromosome
  - influenced by hormone constitution
  - sex-limited inheritance*
  - hen feathering vs. cock feathering*
  - sex-influenced inheritance*
  - heterozygous phenotype depends on gender
  - pattern baldness*

- **Genetic Background and the Environment***
  - penetrance*
  - expressivity*
  - genetic background*
  - position effect
  - heterochromatin
  - temperature effects
  - temperature-sensitive mutations
  - conditional mutations*
  - permissive condition
  - restrictive condition
  - onset of genetic expression*
  - Tay–Sachs disease
  - Lesch–Nyhan syndrome
  - Duchenne muscular dystrophy (DMD)
  - Huntington disease
  - genetic anticipation*

- myotonic dystrophy (DM)
- repeated trinucleotide DNA sequence

- **Extranuclear Inheritance Patterns***
  - extranuclear inheritance*
  - transmission from maternal parent
  - organelle heredity*
  - heteroplasmy*
  - chloroplasts
  - *Mirabilis jalapa*
  - inheritance determined by ovule source*
  - mitochondrial mutations*
  - *poky* in *Neurospora crassa*
  - *petite* in *Saccharomyces cerevisiae*
  - mitochondrial mutations in humans*
  - mtDNA vulnerable to mutations
  - myoclonic epilepsy and ragged red fiber disease (MERRF)
  - tRNA^{Lys}
  - maternal effect*
  - maternal gene products accumulate in egg cytoplasm
  - *Drosophila* embryology*
  - *bicoid* (*bcd*) gene
  - genotype of female parent determines phenotype of offspring

T4.1 Typical monohybrid and dihybrid ratios with the modifications that were covered in detail in the text.

Basic Ratio	Modified Ratio	Explanation
3:1	1:2:1	Incomplete dominance
		Codominance
9:3:3:1	3:6:3:1:2:1	Dominance + incomplete dominance or codominance
	9:3:4	Recessive epistasis
	12:3:1	Dominant epistasis
	9:7	Complementary gene interaction
	9:6:1	Novel phenotypes

F4.1 Illustration of gene interaction, in which products from more than one gene pair influence one characteristic or phenotypic trait.

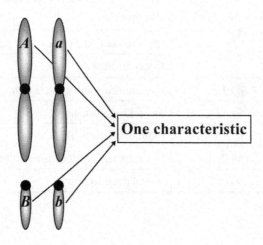

Example: Two gene pairs interact to influence the pigmentation pattern on the shark. Various gene products contribute in a variety of ways to generate a particular pigment pattern.

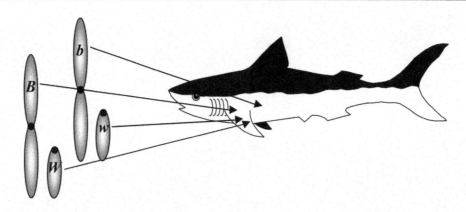

F4.2 Symbolism associated with the wild-type activity of a gene, *M*, that converts precursor A to product B and several possible outcomes of the mutant state: **(A)** wild type, **(B)** too much product, **(C)** too little product, **(D)** no product, **(E)** both products expressed, **(F)** reduced product.

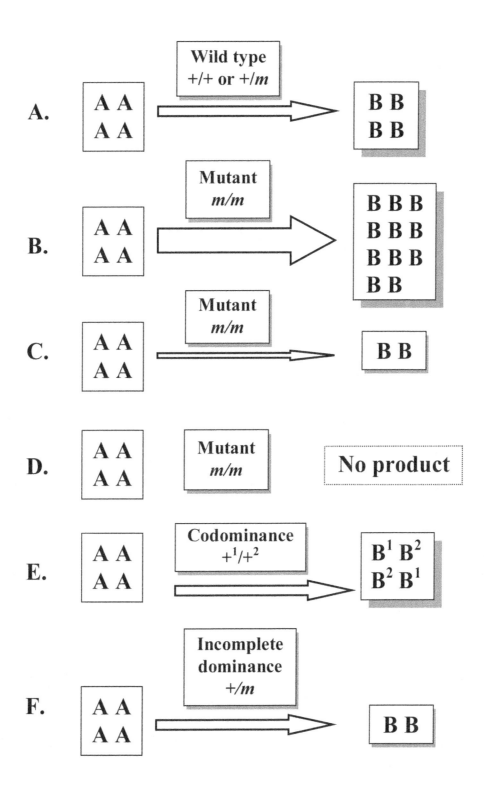

F4.3 Illustration of the common pattern seen in many cases of extranuclear inheritance. The condition of the female (egg) parent has a stronger influence on the phenotype of the offspring than that of the male (sperm/pollen) parent. Reciprocal crosses give different results in offspring.

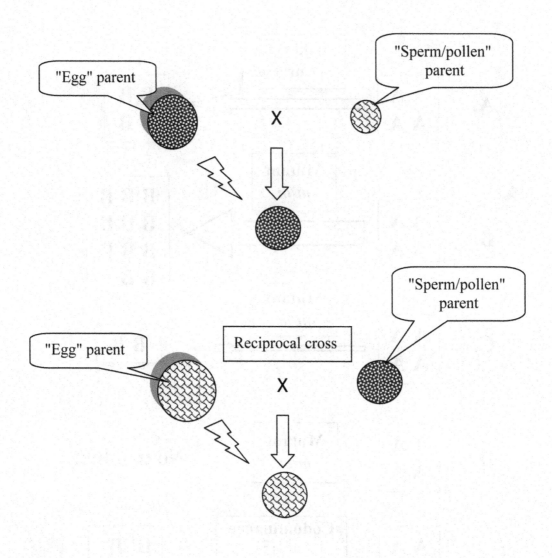

Answers to Now Solve This

4.1 It is important to see that this problem involves multiple alleles, meaning that monohybrid-type ratios are expected, and that there is an order of dominance that will allow certain alleles to be "hidden" in various heterozygotes. As with most genetics problems, one must look at the phenotypes of the offspring to assess the genotypes of the parents.

(a) Parents: sepia × cream

Because both guinea pigs had albino parents, both are heterozygous for the c^a allele.

Cross: $c^k c^a$ × $c^d c^a$ $\Longrightarrow$ 2/4 sepia; 1/4 cream; 1/4 albino

(b) Parents: sepia × cream

Because the sepia parent had an albino parent, it must be $c^k c^a$.

Because the cream guinea pig had two sepia parents

$(c^k c^d \ \times \ c^k c^d \quad$ or $\quad c^k c^d \ \times \ c^k c^a)$,

the cream parent could be either $c^d c^d$ or $c^d c^a$.

Crosses:

if cream parent is homozygous

$c^k c^a \ \times \ c^d c^d$ $\Longrightarrow$ 1/2 sepia; 1/2 cream

OR

if cream parent is heterozygous

$c^k c^a \ \times \ c^d c^a$ $\Longrightarrow$ 1/2 sepia; 1/4 cream; 1/4 albino

(c) Parents: sepia × cream

The sepia guinea pig had two full-color parents, one of which must be Cc^k, and the other of which could be

$Cc^k, \quad Cc^d, \quad$ or $\quad Cc^a$ (*not CC* because sepia could not be produced).

Therefore, there are three possible genotypes for the sepia parent:

$c^k c^k, \quad c^k c^d, \quad$ or $\quad c^k c^a.$

Because the cream guinea pig had two sepia parents

$(c^k c^d \ \times \ c^k c^d \quad$ or $\quad c^k c^d \ \times \ c^k c^a)$,

the cream parent could be either $c^d c^d$ or $c^d c^a$.

Crosses:

$c^k c^k \ \times \ c^d c^d$ $\Longrightarrow$ all sepia

$c^k c^k \ \times \ c^d c^a$ $\Longrightarrow$ all sepia

$c^k c^d \ \times \ c^d c^d$ $\Longrightarrow$ 1/2 sepia; 1/2 cream

$c^k c^d \ \times \ c^d c^a$ $\Longrightarrow$ 1/2 sepia; 1/2 cream

$c^k c^a \ \times \ c^d c^d$ $\Longrightarrow$ 1/2 sepia; 1/2 cream

$c^k c^a \ \times \ c^d c^a$ $\Longrightarrow$ 1/2 sepia; 1/4 cream; 1/4 albino

(d) Parents: sepia × cream

Because the sepia parent had a full-color parent and an albino parent (Cc^k × c^ac^a), it must be c^kc^a.

The cream parent had two full-color parents, one of which must be Cc^d, and the other of which could be Cc^d or Cc^a; therefore, the cream parent could be c^dc^d or c^dc^a.

Crosses:

c^kc^a × c^dc^d ⟹ 1/2 sepia; 1/2 cream

c^kc^a × c^dc^a ⟹ 1/2 sepia; 1/4 cream; 1/4 albino

4.2 Notice that the distribution of observed offspring fits a 9:3:4 ratio quite well. This suggests that two independently assorting gene pairs with epistasis are involved. Assign gene symbols in the usual manner:

A = pigment; a = pigmentless (colorless)

B = purple; b = red

$AaBb$ × $AaBb$

$A-B-$ = purple
$A-bb$ = red
$aaB-$ = colorless
$aabb$ = colorless

One may see this occurring in the following manner, where an "X" indicates a block or missing enzyme in the biochemical pathway:

precursor ---**X**-> cyanidin ---**X**-> purple pigment

          (colorless) *aa*   (red) *bb*

4.3 For all three pedigrees, let *a* represent the mutant gene and *A* represent its normal allele. (Note: this can also be symbolized as X^a and X^A).

(a) This pedigree is consistent with an X-linked recessive trait because the male would contribute an X chromosome carrying the *a* mutation to the *aa* daughter. The mother would have to be heterozygous *Aa* .

(b) This pedigree is consistent with an X-linked recessive trait because the mother could be *Aa* and transmit her *a* allele to her one son (*a*/Y) and her *A* allele to her other son.

(c) This pedigree is not consistent with an X-linked mode of inheritance because the *aa* mother has an *A*/Y son.

Solutions to Problems and Discussion Questions

1. (a) In general, they observed results of crosses that did not produce offspring in typical Mendelian ratios.

(b) Modifications of dihybrid and higher-level ratios indicated that loci were not expressed independently. A 9:3:4 ratio illustrates such a dihybrid modification. The number of gene pairs involved is often determined by correlating the sum of the components of each ratio with the formula 4^n, where n represents the number of gene pairs. For example, a 1:2:1 or 3:1 ratio adds to four (or 4^1), indicating a monohybrid cross. A 9:3:4 or a 12:3:1 ratio adds to 16 (or 4^2), indicating a dihybrid ratio.

(c) Morgan and his colleagues observed that the sex of the parent carrying a mutant allele influenced the results of crosses when compared to a reciprocal cross. When correlated with the sex chromosome differences between males and females, a model placing a gene on the X chromosome was supported.

(d) When a gene is X-linked, ratios from crosses are influenced by which parent contributes a particular allele. When sex-limited or sex-influenced inheritance occurs, the parental source of the allele is irrelevant because the involved genes are autosomal and their expression is dependent on the individual's hormone constitution.

(e) Scientists noted that in some cases, the pattern of inheritance did not follow what was expected of chromosomal genes. With organelle heredity, the cytoplasm carried considerable influence on the phenotype of the progeny, causing reciprocal crosses to give different phenotypic results. In maternal effects, the genotype of the mother, rather than the genotype of the zygote, played a dominant role in determining the phenotype of developing offspring.

2. Your essay should include a description of alleles that do not function independently of each other or that reduce the viability of a class(es) of offspring. With multiple alleles, there are more than two alternatives of a gene at a given locus.

3. (a) In this problem, there is one characteristic (coat color) and three phenotypes: red, white, and roan, with roan being the intermediate between red and white. This suggests that neither allele is dominant.

The data given show that a cross of the "extremes" (red × white) gives roan, suggesting the parents are each homozygous and the offspring heterozygous. The 1:2:1 ratio in the offspring of

$$\text{roan} \quad \times \quad \text{roan}$$

supports the hypothesis of incomplete dominance or codominance as the mode of inheritance.

Symbolism (arbitrarily described here as A and a):

> AA = red
>
> aa = white
>
> Aa = roan

Alternatively, given the absence of dominance, other symbolism (such as C^1C^1 = red; C^2C^2 = white; and C^1C^2 = roan) is often used.

Crosses: It is important at this point that you not be fully dependent on writing out complete Punnett squares for each cross. Begin working these simple problems in your head.

AA × AA ⟹ AA		
aa × aa ⟹ aa		
AA × aa ⟹ Aa		
Aa × Aa ⟶		
1/4 AA; 2/4 Aa; 1/4 aa		

(b) Distinguishing between incomplete dominance and codominance is best done through biochemical examination of the gene product (such as the red pigment molecule). For incomplete dominance, a reduction of pigment levels would be observed. By contrast, for codominance, two alternative pigments would be co-expressed at similar levels.

4. In this problem, remember that individuals with blood type B can have the genotype $I^B I^B$ or $I^B i$ and those with blood type A can have genotypes $I^A I^A$ or $I^A i$.

Male Parent: must be $I^B i$ because his mother is ii and one inherits one homolog (therefore one allele) from each parent.

Female Parent: must be $I^A i$ because her father is $I^B i$ and one inherits one homolog (therefore one allele) from each parent. Her father cannot be $I^B I^B$ and have a daughter of blood type A.

Offspring:

$$I^A i \times I^B i$$

	I^B	i
I^A	$I^A I^B$ (AB)	$I^A i$ (A)
i	$I^B i$ (B)	ii (O)

The expected ratio would be

1(A):1(B):1(AB):1(O).

5. This problem involves one typical (coat color) and one atypical (lethality) characteristic. Often under this condition of two characteristics, we must decide whether the problem involves one or more than one gene pair. Because the genotypes are given here, it is obvious that lethality is associated with expression of the coat color alleles, and therefore one gene pair is involved. This is a monohybrid situation.

$$Pp \times Pp$$
1/4 PP (**lethal**)

2/4 Pp (platinum)

1/4 pp (silver)

Therefore, the ratio of surviving foxes is 2/3 platinum, 1/3 silver. The P allele behaves (1) as a recessive allele in terms of lethality (the P allele is lethal only when homozygous) but (2) as a dominant allele in terms of coat color (platinum, the color encoded by the P allele, is expressed in the heterozygote).

6. Three independently assorting characteristics are being dealt with: flower color (incomplete dominance), flower shape (dominant/recessive), and plant height (dominant/recessive). Establish appropriate gene symbols:

Flower color:
RR = red; Rr = pink; rr = white

Flower shape:
P = personate; p = peloric

Plant height:
D = tall; d = dwarf

The genotype and phenotype of F_1 generation plants will be

$$RRPPDD \times rrppdd$$
$RrPpDd$ (pink, personate, tall)

To determine the proportion of F_2 plants that will be pink, personate, and tall, use *components* of the forked-line method as follows:

2/4 pink $\times$ 3/4 personate $\times$ 3/4 tall = 18/64

7. There are two characteristics: flower color and flower shape. Because pink results from a cross of red and white, one would conclude that flower color is monohybrid with incomplete dominance.

In addition, because personate is seen in the F_1 when personate and peloric are crossed, personate must be dominant to peloric. Results from crosses (c) and (d) verify these conclusions. The appropriate symbols would be as follows:

Flower color:
RR = red; Rr = pink; rr = white

Flower shape:
P = personate; p = peloric

(a)
$$RRpp \times rrPP \implies RrPp$$

(b)
$$RRPP \times rrpp \implies RrPp$$

(c)
$$RrPp \times RRpp \implies \begin{cases} RRPp \\ RRpp \\ RrPp \\ Rrpp \end{cases}$$

(d)
$$RrPp \times rrpp \implies \begin{cases} rrPp \\ rrpp \\ RrPp \\ Rrpp \end{cases}$$

(e) In the cross of the F_1 of (a) to the F_1 of (b), both of which are double heterozygotes, one would expect the following:

RrPp × *RrPp*

1/4 red
    3/4 personate → 3/16 red, personate
    1/4 peloric   → 1/16 red, peloric

2/4 pink
    3/4 personate → 6/16 pink, personate
    1/4 peloric   → 2/16 pink, peloric

1/4 white
    3/4 personate → 3/16 white, personate
    1/4 peloric   → 1/16 white, peloric

8. This is a case of gene interaction (novel phenotypes), whereby mutations that give rise to the yellow and black phenotypes interact to give the cream phenotype (in the double mutants), and of epistasis, whereby the *cc* genotype produces albino.

(a)

all *AaBbCc* ⟹ all gray (*C* allows pigment)

(b)

all *A–B–cc* ⟹ all albino (no color because *cc*)

(c) Use the forked-line method for this portion.

3/4 *A–*
    3/4 *B–*
        1/2 *Cc* ⟹ 9/32 gray
        1/2 *cc* ⟹ 9/32 albino
    1/4 *bb*
        1/2 *Cc* ⟹ 3/32 yellow
        1/2 *cc* ⟹ 3/32 albino

1/4 *aa*
    3/4 *B–*
        1/2 *Cc* ⟹ 3/32 black
        1/2 *cc* ⟹ 3/32 albino
    1/4 *bb*
        1/2 *Cc* ⟹ 1/32 cream
        1/2 *cc* ⟹ 1/32 albino

Combining the phenotypes gives (always count the proportions to see that they add up to 1.0):

16/32 albino
9/32 gray
3/32 yellow
3/32 black
1/32 cream

9. Treat each of the crosses as a series of monohybrid crosses, remembering that albino is epistatic to color and black and yellow interact to give cream.

(a) Because this is a 9:3:3:1 ratio with no albino phenotypes, the parents must each have been double heterozygotes and incapable of producing the *cc* genotype.

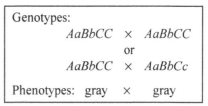

Genotypes:
    AaBbCC × *AaBbCC*
        or
    AaBbCC × *AaBbCc*

Phenotypes: gray × gray

(b) Because there are no black or cream offspring, there are no combinations in the parents that can produce *aa*. The 4/16 proportion of albino indicates that the *C* locus is heterozygous in both parents.

If the parents are

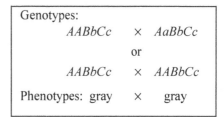

Genotypes:
    AABbCc × *AaBbCc*
        or
    AABbCc × *AABbCc*

Phenotypes: gray × gray

then the results would follow the pattern given.

(c) Notice that 16/64 or 1/4 of the offspring are albino; therefore, the parents are both heterozygous at the *C* locus. Second, notice that without considering the *C* locus, there is a 27:9:9:3 ratio that reduces to a 9:3:3:1 ratio. Given this information, the genotypes and phenotypes must be

Genotypes:
    AaBbCc × *AaBbCc*

Phenotypes: gray × gray

10. First determine the possible genotypes of the parents and the grandfathers. Because the gene is X-linked, the cross will be symbolized with the X chromosomes.

RG = normal vision; *rg* = color-blind

    Wife's father: X^{rg}/Y

    Husband's father: X^{rg}/Y

    Wife: X^{RG}/X^{rg}

    Husband: X^{RG}/Y

The wife must be heterozygous for the *rg* allele (being normal-visioned and having inherited an X^{rg}

from her father), and the husband, because he has normal vision, must be X^{RG}. The fact that the husband's father is color-blind is not relevant because the husband inherited his X chromosome from his mother.

$$X^{RG}/X^{rg} \quad \times \quad X^{RG}/Y$$

$$X^{RG}/X^{RG} \quad = \quad 1/4 \text{ daughter normal}$$

$$X^{RG/}X^{rg} \quad = \quad 1/4 \text{ daughter normal}$$

$$X^{RG}/Y \quad = \quad 1/4 \text{ son normal}$$

$$X^{rg}/Y \quad = \quad 1/4 \text{ son color-blind}$$

Looking at the distribution of offspring:

    (a) 1/4

    (b) 1/2

    (c) 1/4

    (d) zero

11. The mating is $X^{RG}/X^{rg}; I^A/i \times X^{RG}/Y; I^A/i$. Based on the son who is color-blind with blood type O, the mother must have been heterozygous for the *RG* locus, and each parent must have had one copy of the *i* allele. The probability of having a female child is 1/2, that she has normal vision is 1 (because the father's X carries the unaffected allele), and that she has type O blood is 1/4. The final product of the independent probabilities is

$$1/2 \quad \times \quad 1 \quad \times \quad 1/4 \quad = \quad 1/8$$

12. Seeing the different distribution between males and females, one might consider sex-influenced inheritance as a model and have males more likely to express bearded and females more likely to express beardless in the heterozygote. This situation is similar to pattern baldness in humans. Consider two alleles that are autosomal and let

    BB = beardless in both sexes
    Bb = beardless in females
    Bb = bearded in males
    bb = bearded in both sexes

P$_1$: female: *bb* (bearded) × male: *BB* (beardless)

F$_1$: *Bb* = males bearded; female beardless

Because half of the offspring are males and half are females, one could, for clarity, rewrite the F$_2$ as:

	1/2 males	1/2 females
1/4 *BB*	1/8 beardless	1/8 beardless
2/4 *Bb*	2/8 bearded	2/8 beardless
1/4 *bb*	1/8 bearded	1/8 bearded

One could test this model by crossing F$_1$ (heterozygous) beardless females with bearded (homozygous) males. Comparing these results with the reciprocal cross would support the model if the distributions of sexes with phenotypes were the same in both crosses.

13. The tortoiseshell condition is caused by the phenomenon of dosage compensation, whereby one of the two X chromosomes is randomly inactivated in mammalian females. Once inactivated, all cells descending from a given cell will have the same X chromosome inactive. A tortoiseshell female is *Bb* and when crossed with a *B*Y male produces the following offspring:

$$Bb \quad \times \quad BY$$

females: *BB* (black)
                 Bb (tortoiseshell)

males: *B*Y (black)
             *b*Y (orange)

From this information, it would seem impossible to get a tortoiseshell male; however, rare nondisjunction in the female or male parent can produce a tortoiseshell male with the *Bb*Y genotype.

14. Symbolism: Normal wing margins = X^+ scalloped = X^{sd}

(a)

P$_1$:	$X^{sd}/X^{sd} \times X^+/Y$
F$_1$:	1/2 X^+/X^{sd} (female, normal)
	1/2 X^{sd}/Y (male, scalloped)
F$_2$:	1/4 X^+/X^{sd} (female, normal)
	1/4 X^{sd}/X^{sd} (female, scalloped)
	1/4 X^+/Y (male, normal)
	1/4 X^{sd}/Y (male, scalloped)

(b)

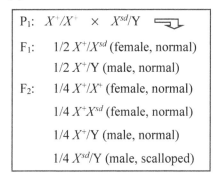

P_1: X^+/X^+ × X^{sd}/Y

F_1: 1/2 X^+/X^{sd} (female, normal)

  1/2 X^+/Y (male, normal)

F_2: 1/4 X^+/X^+ (female, normal)

  1/4 X^+X^{sd} (female, normal)

  1/4 X^+/Y (male, normal)

  1/4 X^{sd}/Y (male, scalloped)

If the *scalloped* gene were not X-linked, then all of the F_1 offspring would be wild type (phenotypically) and a 3:1 ratio of normal to scalloped would occur among all offspring in the F_2, regardless of sex.

15. Assuming that the parents are homozygous, the crosses would be as follows. Notice that the X symbol may remain to remind us that the *sd* gene is on the X chromosome. It is extremely important to account for both the mutant genes and each of their wild-type alleles.

P_1: X^{sd}/X^{sd}; e^+/e^+ × X^+/Y; e/e

F_1: 1/2 X^+/X^{sd}; e^+/e (female, normal wings, normal body)

  1/2 X^{sd}/Y; e^+/e (male, scalloped wings, normal body)

F_2:

	X^+e^+	X^+e	$X^{sd}e^+$	$X^{sd}e$
$X^{sd}e^+$				
$X^{sd}e$		Fill in box		
Ye^+		on your own.		
Ye				

Phenotypes:

3/16 female with normal wings and body

3/16 male with normal wings and body

1/16 ebony female with normal wings

1/16 ebony male with normal wings

3/16 scalloped female with normal body

3/16 scalloped male with normal body

1/16 scalloped, ebony female

1/16 scalloped, ebony male

Forked-line method:

P_1: X^{sd}/X^{sd}; e^+/e^+ × X^+/Y; e/e

F_1: 1/2 X^+/X^{sd}; e^+/e (female, normal)

  1/2 X^{sd}/Y; e^+/e (male, scalloped)

F_2:

	Wings	Color	
1/4	female, normal	3/4 normal	3/16
		1/4 ebony	1/16
1/4	female, scalloped	3/4 normal	3/16
		1/4 ebony	1/16
1/4	males, normal	3/4 normal	3/16
		1/4 ebony	1/16
1/4	male, scalloped	3/4 normal	3/16
		1/4 ebony	1/16

16. It is extremely important to account for both the mutant genes and each of their wild-type alleles.

Symbolism: $X^+/-$; $+/- $ = wild type

  X^v/X^v; $+/-$ or X^v/Y; $+/-$ = vermillion

  $X^+/-$; bw/bw = brown

  X^v/X^v; bw/bw or X^v/Y; bw/bw = white

(a)

P_1: X^vX^v; $+/+$ × X^+/Y; bw/bw

F_1: 1/2 X^+X^v; $+/bw$ (female, normal)

  1/2 X^v/Y; $+/bw$ (male, vermilion)

F_2:

Eye color (X)   Eye color (autosomal)

1/4	female, normal	3/4 normal	3/16
		1/4 brown	1/16
1/4	female, vermilion	3/4 normal	3/16
		1/4 brown	1/16
1/4	males, normal	3/4 normal	3/16
		1/4 brown	1/16
1/4	male, vermilion	3/4 normal	3/16
		1/4 brown	1/16

3/16 = female, normal

1/16 = female, brown eyes

3/16 = female, vermilion eyes

1/16 = female, white eyes ***(Continue on next page)***

3/16 = male, normal

1/16 = male, brown eyes

3/16 = male, vermilion eyes

1/16 = male, white eyes

(b)

P₁: X^+X^+; *bw/bw* × X^vY; +/+

F₁: 1/2 X^+X^v; +/*bw* (female, normal)
1/2 X^+/Y; +/*bw* (male, normal)

F_2:

Eye color (X)		Eye color (autosomal)	
2/4	female, normal	3/4 normal	6/16
		1/4 brown	2/16
1/4	male, normal	3/4 normal	3/16
		1/4 brown	1/16
1/4	male, vermilion	3/4 normal	3/16
		1/4 brown	1/16

6/16 = female, normal

2/16 = female, brown eyes

3/16 = male, normal

1/16 = male, brown eyes

3/16 = male, vermilion eyes

1/16 = male, white eyes

(c)

P_1: X^vX^v; *bw/bw* × X^+/Y; +/+

F_1: 1/2 X^+X^v; +/*bw* (female, normal)
1/2 X^v/Y; +/*bw* (male, vermilion)

F_2: The F_2 progeny for this cross will be identical to that for the cross in (a), since the genotypes of the F_1 flies are identical in both questions.

17. The key to dealing with this problem is seeing that there are two genotypes that can produce the sandy phenotype. Notice that in cross 1, crossing sandy with sandy gives an F_1 with the all-red phenotype. Because the problem states that all of the strains are true-breeding, there is likely some sort of complementation between the two sandy strains to give the all-red F_1 in cross 1. If you start out with that premise and assign the following genotypic possibilities, all the data fall into place:

A–B– = red
A–bb or *aaB–* = sandy
aabb = white

For the lost data in crosses 1 and 4, use the following:

Cross 1: *aaBB* × *AAbb*

F_1: *AaBb*

F_2:

9/16 = *A–B–*(red)
6/16 { 3/16 = *A–bb* (sandy)
3/16 = *aaB–* (sandy)
1/16 = *aabb* (white)

Cross 4: *aabb* × *AABB*

F_1: *AaBb*

F_2:

9/16 = *A–B–*(red)
6/16 { 3/16 = *A–bb* (sandy)
3/16 = *aaB–*(sandy)
1/16 = *aabb* (white)

18. (a) The denominator in the ratios is 64 (or 4^3), which suggests that there are three independently assorting gene pairs operating in this problem. Because there are only two characteristics (eye color and croaking), however, one might hypothesize that two gene pairs are involved in the inheritance of one trait, whereas one gene pair is involved in the other.

(b) The 48:16 (or 3:1) ratio of utterers to mutterers indicates that croaking is due to one (dominant/recessive) gene pair. Furthermore, the 36:16:12 (or 9:4:3) ratio of blue to green to purple eye color indicates that eye color is due to two gene pairs that interact (specifically, by recessive epistasis).

(c) Symbolism:

Croaking: *R–* = utterer; *rr* = mutterer

Eye color: Because the most frequent phenotype is blue eye, let *A–B–*represent 9/16 genotypes. For the purple class, a 3/16 group uses the *A–bb* genotypes. The 4/16 class (green) would be the *aaB–*and the *aabb* groups.

Therefore, the genotypes are:
P_1: *AAbbRR* x *aaBBrr*
F_1: *AaBbRr*
F_2: See the genotypes listed in the "Eye color" paragraph immediately preceding

(d) The cross involving a true-breeding blue-eyed, mutterer frog and a true-breeding purple-eyed, utterer frog would have the genotypes

$$AABBrr \quad \times \quad AAbbRR.$$

All F_1 individuals would have a genotype of $AABbRr$, and would be blue-eyed utterers. The F_2 would follow a pattern of a 9:3:3:1 ratio because of homozygosity for the A locus and heterozygosity for both the B and R loci.

9/16 AAB–R– = blue-eyed, utterer

3/16 AAB–rr = blue-eyed, mutterer

3/16 $AAbbR$–= purple-eyed, utterer

1/16 $AAbbrr$ = purple-eyed, mutterer

19. Suggested approach to these types of problems: Take each characteristic individually, then build the complete genotypes. Eye color: (1) Both parents have purple eyes, so the B locus would have the bb genotype for each. (2) The F_2 ratio of purple-eyed to green-eyed frogs is 3:1; therefore, expect the parents to be heterozygous for the A locus. Croaking: Because the ratio of utterers to mutterers is also 3:1, expect both parents to be heterozygous at the R locus. Putting this information together, both parents would have the genotype $AabbRr$.

20. The denominator in the ratios is 16, which suggests that two independently assorting gene pairs interact to produce coat color. The data for the cross between F_1 individuals shows that a 12:3:1 ratio is obtained, a clear sign that dominant epistasis has modified a typical 9:3:3:1 ratio. In this case, cattle in one of the 3/16 classes have the same phenotype as cattle in the 9/16 class.

Because the 9/16 class typically takes the genotype of A–B–, it seems reasonable to think of the following genotypic classifications:

A–B– = solid white (9/16)

aaB– = solid white (3/16)

A–bb = black-and-white spotted (3/16)

$aabb$ = solid black (1/16)

One could obtain $AAbb$ true-breeding black-and-white spotted cattle.

21. (a, b) The condition cannot be dominant because it appears in the offspring (II-3 and II-4) of unaffected parents in the first two families. In the second cross, the father is not shaded, yet the daughter (II-4) is. Therefore, X-linked recessive does not fit. If the condition is recessive, then it must be *autosomal*.

(c) II-1 = AA or Aa

II-6 = AA or Aa

II-9 = Aa

22. First, look for familiar ratios that will inform you as to the general mode of inheritance. Notice that the last cross (h) gives a 9:4:3 ratio, which is typical of recessive epistasis. From this information, one can develop a model to account for the results given. Let the B locus determine whether color is expressed (genotypes B–) or not expressed (genotype bb = golden). And, when there is at least one dominant allele at the B locus, let the A locus determine color: A– = black and aa = brown.

Symbolism:

A–B– = black

A–bb = golden (due to the bb genotype)

$aabb$ = golden (due to the bb genotype)

aaB– = brown

To solve this type of problem, first determine the parental genotypes at the B locus (ask whether any progeny are golden and in what proportion), then determine the genotypes at the A locus based on the ratio of black to brown.

(a) AAB– $\times$ $aaBB$ or $AABB \times aaB$–. One or both parents must be homozygous dominant at the B locus, and the black parent must be homozygous dominant at the A locus.

(b) AaB–$\times$ $aaBB$ or $AaBB \times aaB$–. Notice that both parents cannot be Bb.

(c) $AABb \times aaBb$. Both parents must be heterozygous at the B locus to produce 1/4 golden progeny.

(d) $AABB \times$ —bb or $AaBB \times AAbb$.

(e) $AaBb \times Aabb$.

(f) $AaBb \times aabb$

(g) $aaBb \times aaBb$

(h) $AaBb \times AaBb$

Those genotypes that will breed true will be as follows:

black = $AABB$

golden = all (Because all are genotypically bb.)

brown = $aaBB$

23. The test for allelism is made by crossing the various mutant strains. If the resulting offspring are mutant, then the mutations are allelic (same gene). If the offspring are wild type, then the mutations are not allelic (different genes) and complementation is occurring. In cross 1, all of the offspring are wild type, indicating that *r1* and *r2* are complementing and therefore not allelic. In cross 2, all of the offspring have tan eyes, indicating that the mutations are allelic. Because mutations *r1* and *r3* are in the same gene and *r1* and *r2* are not, the cross *r2* × *r3* should be complementing and will result in progeny with wild-type eyes; that is, *r2* and *r3* are in different genes.

24. (a) This question involves the *cremello* locus, which modifies (dilutes) the expression of coat color, making it lighter. The genotype at the coat color locus is the same for all these horses, so we will consider the genotype only at the *cremello* locus. This is a case of incomplete dominance in which matings between heterozygotes (palomino) produce a typical 1:2:1 F_2 ratio (see the third cross). Therefore, one can set the following symbols:

CC = chestnut

$C^{CR} C^{CR}$ = cremello

$C\ C^{CR}$ = palomino

(b) The F_1 resulting from matings between cremello and chestnut horses would be expected to be all palomino. The F_2 would be expected to fall in a 1:2:1 ratio as in the third cross in part **(a)**.

25. This is a case in which recessive epistasis (from *cc*) results in a "masking" of genes at the *A* locus. In this case, there will be modifications of typical 9:3:3:1 and 1:1:1:1 ratios because of gene interactions.

(a) In a cross of

$AACC$ × *aacc*

the offspring are all *AaCc* (agouti) because the *C* allele allows pigment to be deposited in the hair, and when it is, it will be agouti. F_2 offspring would have the following "simplified" genotypes with the corresponding phenotypes:

A–C– = 9/16 (agouti)

A–cc = 3/16 (colorless due to the *cc* genotype)

aaC– = 3/16 (black)

aacc = 1/16 (colorless due to the *cc* genotype)

The two colorless classes are phenotypically indistinguishable; therefore, the final ratio is 9:3:4.

(b) Results of crosses of female agouti

(*A–C–*) × *aacc* (males)

are given in three groups:

(1) To produce equivalent numbers of agouti and colorless offspring, the female parent must have been *AACc* so that half of the offspring are able to deposit pigment because of *C*, and when they do, they are all agouti (having received only *A* from the female parent).

(2) To produce an even number of agouti and black offspring, the mother must have been *Aa,* and because no colorless offspring were produced, the female must have been *CC*. Her genotype must have been *AaCC*.

(3) Notice that half of the offspring are colorless; therefore, the female must have been *Cc*. Half of the pigmented offspring are black and half are agouti; therefore, the female must have been *Aa*. Overall, the *AaCc* genotype is likely.

26. First, make certain that you understand the genetics of all of the gene pairs being described in the problem. The ABO system involves multiple alleles, codominance, and dominance. The MN system has two alleles that are codominant. The easiest way to approach these types of problems is to consider those gene pairs that produce a low number of options in the offspring. Notice in cross 1 that there are two options in the offspring for the ABO system (types A and O), but only one option for the MN system (type MN). By looking at the most restrictive classes, one can determine that option (c) is the only one that is both MN and O. The remainder of the combinations can be determined using the same logic.

Cross 1 = (c)

Cross 2 = (d)

Cross 3 = (b)

Cross 4 = (e)

Cross 5 = (a)

This is the only set of matches possible, given that each of the five matings resulted in one of the five offspring shown.

27. Passage of X-linked genes typically occurs from carrier mother to affected son. The fact that the father in couple 2 has hemophilia would not predispose his son to hemophilia. The first couple has no valid claim.

28. The clue to the solution comes from the description of the Dexter breed: They are not true-breeding and are, therefore, always heterozygous. Coupled with this, their observed low fertility rates indicate that the homozygous genotype type is lethal. Furthermore, the F_1 results show that the Kerry breed is homozygous recessive. Polled is caused by an independently assorting dominant allele, whereas horned is caused by the recessive allele to polled.

29. In cases of extranuclear inheritance, the phenotype is determined by the nuclear (maternal effect) or cytoplasmic (organelle) condition of the parent (usually maternal) that contributes the bulk of the cytoplasm to the offspring.

(a) In Mendelian (chromosomal) inheritance, it does not matter which parent contributes a mutant allele to the offspring – reciprocal crosses produce the same results in both the F_1 and F_2 generations. By contrast, in extranuclear inheritance, both parents do not contribute to the characteristics of the offspring. Instead, the pattern of inheritance is more often from only one parent to the offspring. Standard Mendelian ratios (3:1) are usually not present. In general, the results of reciprocal crosses differ.
See F4.3 in this handbook.

> *Female mutant × male wild*
>
> all offspring mutant
>
> _____
>
> *Female wild × male mutant*
>
> all offspring wild

(b) In sex-linked inheritance, the pattern is often from carrier (unaffected) mother to son. Patterns of extranuclear inheritance are often not influenced by the sex of the offspring.

30. Developmental phenomena that occur early are more likely to be under maternal influence than those occurring late. Anterior/posterior and dorsal/ventral orientations are among the earliest to be established, and organisms whose study is experimentally and/or genetically approachable often show considerable maternal influence. Maternal effect genes encode products that are not carried over for more than one generation, unlike organelle heredity. Crosses that

illustrate the transient nature of a maternal effect could include the following.

Female Aa × male aa → all offspring of the A phenotype (even though half of the offspring are genotypically aa).

From these progeny, take a female that is genotypically aa despite having an A phenotype and conduct the following mating: aa × male Aa. All offspring from this cross might* be of the a phenotype because all of the offspring will reflect the *genotype* of the mother, not her *phenotype*. (*Note that in actual practice, the results of this cross would give a typical 1:1 ratio because the mother might be either Aa or aa.) This cross illustrates that maternal effects last for only one generation. Had the phenotype been inherited through organelle heredity, the maternal phenotype would have persisted in each generation.

31. **(a)** The presence of bcd^-/bcd^- males can be explained by the maternal effect: Mothers were bcd^+/bcd^- and were able to provide the bicoid protein to the egg.

(b) The cross

   female bcd^+/bcd^- × male bcd^-/bcd^-

will produce an F_1 with normal embryogenesis because heterozygous mothers were able to supply the bicoid protein to all eggs. In the F_2, any cross having bcd^+/bcd^- mothers will produce progeny with normal embryogenesis. By contrast, any cross involving homozygous bcd^-/bcd^- mothers will yield progeny that fail to complete embryogenesis.

32. (a) The reduced ratio is 12 white, 3 orange, and 1 brown, therefore dominant epistasis is occurring. The genotypes for a dihybrid cross are as follows:

F_1: *AaBb*

F_2: 12 white *A–B–* or *aaB–*

   3 orange *A–bb*

   1 brown *aabb*

(b) To solve the problem for three gene pairs, direct your attention to text Figure 3.9, which shows the phenotype ratios for a trihybrid cross and see what you can come up with.

33. These data are consistent with the occurrence of gene interaction with the absence of complete dominance. The different phenotypes result from heterozygous- versus homozygous-dominant states.

(For example, in the following solution, *AaBB* gives magenta, whereas *AaBb* gives rose.) One possible explanation that accounts for these results follows.

The true-breeding parents have the following genotypes:

> *aabb* = crimson
>
> *AABB* = white

The F_1 consists of *AaBb* genotypes with a rose phenotype.

In the F_2, the following genotypes correspond to the given phenotypes:

AA— = white 4/16

AaBB = magenta 2/16

AaBb = rose 4/16

Aabb = orange 2/16

aaBB = yellow 1/16

aaBb = pale yellow 2/16

aabb = crimson 1/16

34. Beatrice, Alice of Hesse, and Alice of Athlone are carriers. There is a 1/2 chance that Princess Irene is a carrier.

Chapter 5: Sex Determination and Sex Chromosomes

Concept Areas	Corresponding Problems
Sex Chromosomes	1, 2, 3, 10, 13, 14, 15, 16, 17, 21, 23, 24, 26
Nondisjunction	9, 13, 14, 17, 21
Sex Determination	1, 3, 4, 5, 6, 8, 11, 15, 23, 25, 26, 27
Sexual Differentiation	4, 5, 12, 25, 26, 27
Dosage Compensation	1, 7, 16, 17, 18, 19, 20, 21, 22

Structures and Processes Checklist—Significant items that deserve special attention are identified with a "*".

(Check topic when mastered–provide examples where appropriate–understand the context of each entry)

○ **Overview**

    ○ sexual differentiation

    ○ heteromorphic chromosomes

    ○ sex chromosomes*

    ○ sex determination

○ **X and Y Chromosomes***

    ○ X-body

    ○ heterochromosome

    ○ *Protenor* mode of sex determination*

    ○ XX/XO

    ○ *Lygaeus* mode of sex determination*

    ○ Y chromosome

    ○ XX/XY

    ○ heterogametic sex*

    ○ homogametic sex*

    ○ ZZ/ZW*

○ **Male Determination in Humans***

    ○ 23 chromosome pairs

    ○ X, Y chromosomes

    ○ Y chromosome determines maleness

    ○ Klinefelter syndrome (47,XXY)

    ○ Turner syndrome (45,X)

    ○ nondisjunction*

    ○ 48,XXXY

    ○ 48,XXYY

    ○ 49,XXXXY

    ○ 49,XXXYY

    ○ mosaics*

    ○ 45,X/46,XY

    ○ 45,X/46,XX

    ○ 47,XXX

    ○ triplo-X

    ○ 48,XXXX

    ○ 49,XXXXX

- 47,XYY*
- sexual differentiation in humans*
- gonadal (genital) ridges
- cortex and medulla
- bipotential gonads*
- presence/absence of Y chromosome*
- Y chromosome and maleness*
- pseudoautosomal regions (PARs)
- male-specific region of the Y (MSY)*
- *sex-determining region Y (SRY)** gene
- testis-determining factor (TDF)*
- transgenic mice
- transcription factor
- master switch
- *SOX9* gene
- paternal age effects (PAE)

- **Ratio of Males to Females***
  - potential for equal proportions
  - sex ratio*
  - primary sex ratio (PSR)
  - secondary sex ratio

- **Dosage Compensation in Mammals**
  - genetic dosage difference
  - X-linked genes
  - dosage compensation*
  - sex chromatin body, or Barr body
  - *N*–1 rule*

- Lyon hypothesis*
- X-linked coat color genes *
- clone
- *glucose-6-phosphate dehydrogenase (G6PD)* gene*
- red-green color blindness
- heterozygous females are mosaics
- mechanism of inactivation*
- imprinting*
- epigenetics
- X-inactivation center (*Xic*)*
- expressed on inactivated X
- *X-inactive specific transcript (XIST)* gene

- **Sex Determination in *Drosophila* and *C. elegans***
  - no role for Y chromosome
  - *Drosophila melanogaster*
  - Calvin Bridges
  - nondisjunction studies*
  - XXY and XO flies
  - progeny of triploid (3*n*) females*
  - metafemales
  - metamales
  - intersexes
  - genic balance theory*
  - X:A ratio*
  - *transformer (tra)* gene
  - *Sex-lethal (Sxl)* gene
  - master switch

- *doublesex* (*dsx*) gene
- RNA splicing
- alternative splicing
- *Caenorhabditis elegans*
- approximately 1000 cells
- precise lineage
- hermaphrodites (XX)
- males (XO)

- **Sex Determination in Reptiles***
  - temperature-dependent sex determination (TSD)*
  - three distinct patterns
  - pivotal temperature (T_p)
  - aromatase
  - sex steroids

Answers to Now Solve This

5.1 (a) Something is missing from the male-determining system of sex determination at the level of the genes, gene products, or receptors, and so on and the loss is correlated with CMD1.

(b) The *SOX9* gene, or its product, is probably involved in male development. Perhaps it is activated by *SRY*, which would explain the lack of expression in development of female gonads.

(c) There is probably some evolutionary relationship between the *SOX9* gene and *SRY*. There is considerable evidence that many other genes and pseudogenes are also homologous to *SRY*.

(d) Normal female sexual development does not require the *SOX9* gene or gene product(s).

5.2 Because of X chromosome inactivation in mammals, scientists would be interested in determining whether the nucleus taken from Rainbow (donor) would continue to show such inactivation. The white patches of CC are due to an autosomal gene *S* for white spotting that prevents pigment formation in the cell lineages in which it is expressed. Homozygous *SS* cats have more white than heterozygous *Ss* cats, and there is no absolute pattern of patches due to the *S* allele. Therefore, the distribution of white patches on CC would be expected to differ from that in Rainbow. Furthermore, the gene that produces orange or black coat colors are X-linked. Calico cats like Rainbow are heterozygous for this gene and express patches of orange or black depending on which X chromosome is inactivated in a particular cell. The somatic nucleus from which CC was created contained an inactivated X chromosome. If it *remained inactivated*, she would express only the allele on the active X chromosome. As a result, her patches would be either black or orange. However, if the inactive X in the donor nucleus *reverted to an active state* in the zygote and then went through random inactivation, CC would develop as a calico with both orange and black patches of different size and distribution than seen in Rainbow. In either case, CC would have a different patch pattern from that of her genetic mother based on random X-inactivation alone.

Chapter 5 Sex Determination and Sex Chromosomes

Solutions to Problems and Discussion Questions

1. (a) Supported by the discovery of sex chromosome aneuploids (XO, XXY, for example), presence or absence of a Y chromosome has been shown to be fundamental in sex determination in humans.

(b) In 1948, consensus data of the sex of embryos and fetuses recovered from miscarriages and abortions showed that fetal mortality was higher for males than for females. Based on this finding and the measured secondary sex ratio, the primary sex ratio (PSR) was estimated at 1.079. In 2015, one key parameter used was direct sex assessment of 3- and 6-day-old embryos that were conceived using assisted reproductive technologies. This study concluded that the PSR is about equal between males and females and that prenatal mortality is higher for females than for males.

(c) The most direct evidence in support of random inactivation of either X chromosome in an XX cell came from experiments using electrophoretic variants of the products of the *G6PD* locus. Such studies, coupled with mosaic coat patterns in mammals, support the random inactivation hypothesis.

(d) In mammals, a XO individual develops as a female whereas, in *Drosophila*, an XO individual develops as a male. Likewise, XXY mammals are male whereas XXY fruit flies are female. Calvin Bridges studied a number of chromosomal compositions in *Drosophila* and determined that the critical factor in sex determination is the ratio of X chromosomes to the number of haploid sets of autosomes.

2. Your essay should include various aspects of sex chromosomes that contain genes responsible for sex determination. Mention should also be made of those organisms in which autosomes play a role in concert with the sex chromosomes.

3. (a) The term *homomorphic* refers to the situation in which both of the sex chromosomes have the same form. The term *heteromorphic* refers to the condition in many organisms in which there are two different forms (morphs) of chromosomes, such as X and Y.

(b) In a heteromorphic organism, the *homogametic sex* is the one that bears two of the same type of sex chromosome (such as XX females) and who, therefore produce gametes that all carry that type of sex chromosome. Individuals of the *heterogametic sex* are those that bear two types of sex chromosomes (such as XY males) and who, therefore, produce two different types of gametes.

4. In sexual determination, genes signal developmental pathways whereby the sexes are generated. Sexual differentiation is the complex set of responses by cells, tissues, and organs to those genetic signals.

5. The *Protenor* form of sex determination involves the XX/XO condition, whereby sex is determined by the presence or absence of a chromosome. The *Lygaeus* mode, by contrast, involves the XX/XY condition, where either the Y chromosome or the genic balance between the number of X chromosomes and sets of autosomes determines sex.

6. In *Drosophila,* sex is determined by the balance between the number of X chromosomes and the number of haploid sets of autosomes. The Y chromosome is not involved in sex determination. By contrast, in humans there is a small region on the Y chromosome (the "master switch" gene, *SRY*) that determines maleness.

7. Mammals possess a system of X chromosome inactivation whereby one of the two X chromosomes in females becomes a chromatin body or Barr body. If one of the two X chromosomes is randomly inactivated, the dosage of genetic information is more or less equivalent in males (XY) and females (XX).

8. In humans, it was observed that individuals with the 47,XXY complement are males, whereas those with 45,XO are females. Thus, the Y chromosome was deduced as male determining in humans—specifically, the sex-determining region (*SRY*). *SRY* encodes a product called the testis-determining factor (TDF), which causes the undifferentiated gonadal tissue to form testes. This conclusion has been supported by two observations: (1) that individuals with the 47,XXY complement are males, while 45,XO produces females, and (2) that individuals who are XX but with the *SRY* gene translocated to one X chromosome develop as males and XY individuals with the *SRY* gene deleted or nonfunctional are phenotypically female. By contrast, XO *Drosophila* are males, and XXY individuals are female. Studies on the offspring of triploid females led to the realization that it is the balance between the number of X chromosomes and the number of haploid sets of autosomes that determines sex in *Drosophila*.

9. Failure of the two X homologues to separate in meiosis I will lead to two meiotic products each with two X chromosomes and two products with no X chromosomes. One of these products will be the oocyte. Similarly, failure of two sister chromatids of one of the

X homologues to separate in meiosis II will lead to two normal products, one product with two X chromosomes, and one product with no X chromosome. One of these will be the oocyte. Fertilization of an oocyte with two X chromosomes by a Y-bearing sperm cell would produce XXY Klinefelter syndrome. Fertilization of an oocyte lacking an X chromosome by a normal X-bearing sperm will produce XO Turner syndrome.

10. (a) female $X^{rw}Y$ $\times$ male X^+X^+

F₁:	females:	all X^+Y (normal)
	males:	all $X^{rw}X^+$ (normal)

F₂:	females:	1/2 X^+Y (normal)
		1/2 $X^{rw}Y$ (reduced wing)
	males:	1/2 $X^{rw}X^+$ (normal)
		1/2 X^+X^+ (normal)

(b) female $X^{rw}X^{rw}$ $\times$ male X^+Y

F₁:	females:	all $X^{rw}X^+$ (normal)
	males:	all $X^{rw}Y$ (reduced wing)

F₂:	females:	1/2 $X^{rw}X^+$ (normal)
		1/2 $X^{rw}X^{rw}$ (reduced wing)
	males:	1/2 X^+Y (normal)
		1/2 $X^{rw}Y$ (reduced wing)

11. No. Because the presence of the Y chromosome (*Lygaeus* mode) versus absence of a second sex chromosome (*Protenor* mode) cannot be detected in these crosses, there is no way to distinguish the two modes of sex determination. The crosses would have the same predicted phenotypic outcomes if applying either the XX/XO or XX/XY condition.

12. In the female, the absence of a Y chromosome leads to the development of ovaries. In the male, however, the presence of the Y chromosome initiates development of testes, which secrete hormones that support continued male sexual differentiation. In addition, they inhibit female differentiation. Because male and female calves share a common placenta, they also share the hormonal factors carried in blood. The development of the female calf is affected in a way that suppresses female organ development and enhances masculinization, resulting in a freemartin.

13. In the cross described in the problem ($X^{w\wedge}X^wY \times X^mY$), one would see daughters with the white-eye phenotype and normal wings ($X^{w\wedge}X^wY$) and sons with the miniature-wing phenotype and red eyes (X^mY). This is because attached-X chromosomes have a mother-to-daughter inheritance and the father's X is transferred to the son. Metafemales (in this cross, $X^{w\wedge}X^wX^m$) typically die as third-instar larvae. The rare ones that survive to

adulthood would have wild-type eye color and normal wings. The YY zygotes fail to develop into larvae.

14. If some male offspring had white eyes and normal wings (genotypically X^wY) and some female offspring were wild type (genotypically $X^{w+}X^{+m}$), one might suspect that the attached-X had become unattached.

15. This situation would be detrimental to sex-determining mechanisms. Synapsis of chromosomes in meiotic tissue is often accompanied by crossing over. If sex-determining loci on the Y chromosome were transferred, through crossing over, to the X chromosome, genetically XX individuals could develop at least partially as males.

16. A *Barr body* is an X chromosome that is considered to be genetically inactive. It is seen as a differentially staining chromosome at the periphery in some interphase nuclei of mammals with two or more X chromosomes. There will be one fewer Barr body than the number of X chromosomes.

17. There is a simple formula for determining the number of Barr bodies in a given cell: $N - 1$, where N is the number of X chromosomes.

Klinefelter syndrome (XXY)	= 1
Turner syndrome (XO)	= 0
47,XYY	= 0
47,XXX	= 2
48,XXXX	= 3

18. The *Lyon hypothesis* states that the inactivation of the X chromosome occurs at random early in embryonic development in mammals. Inactivated X chromosomes are "marked" in some way, such that all clonally related cells have the same X chromosome inactivated.

19. Unless other markers, cytological or molecular, are available, one cannot test the Lyon hypothesis with homozygous X-linked genes. The test requires heterozygosity for identification of allelic alternatives to see differences in X chromosome activity.

20. Females may display mosaic retinas with patches of defective color perception. Under these conditions, their color vision may be influenced.

21. Phenotypic mosaicism is dependent on the heterozygous condition of genes on the two X chromosomes. Dosage compensation and the formation of Barr bodies occur only when there are two or more X chromosomes. Females normally have two X chromosomes, while males normally have only one X chromosome; therefore, such mosaicism cannot occur in males. There are rare cases of male calico and tortoiseshell cats that are XXY.

22. Autosomal genes in males and females are expressed from two copies (identical or similar) of each gene. X-linked genes may also be required for normal cellular and organismic processes that function in both sexes. Because males carry only a single copy of the X chromosome, the output of these genes must be balanced in some manner, even if the gene products have nothing to do with sex determination or sex differentiation.

23. Because there is a region of synapsis close to the *Sry*-containing section on the Y chromosome, crossing over in this region would generate XY translocations that would lead to the condition described.

24. Because of the homology between the *red* and *green* genes, the possibility exists for an irregular synapsis (see the following figure) that, following crossing over, would give a chromosome with only one (*green*) of the duplicated genes. When this X chromosome combines with the normal Y chromosome, the son's phenotype can be explained.
Normal synapsis:

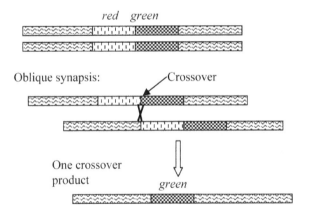

25. The presence of the Y chromosome provides a factor or factors that lead to the initial specification of maleness and the formation of testes. Subsequent expression of secondary sex characteristics must be dependent on the interaction between the gene product of the normal X-linked *Tfm* allele with testosterone. Without such interaction, differentiation takes the female path. It is likely that the *Tfm* gene product is a testosterone (androgen) receptor. To test whether this is the case, one could create engineered mice in which the *Tfm* gene has been replaced by a wild-type copy of a rat androgen receptor gene. If the hypothesis is correct, XY mice that carry the rat gene should develop as normal males.

26. One can conclude that the general architecture of sex determination in fowl is comparable to that in humans (the presence of heteromorphic chromosomes and a sex-determining gene, plus the need for dosage compensation); however, the specific mechanism is somewhat reversed. In chickens, the sex-determining gene, *DMRT1*, is located on the Z chromosome, which is found in both males and females. By contrast, in humans the *SRY* gene is located on the male-specific chromosome. The gene dosage to induce testis development also differs: A single copy of *SRY* is sufficient, whereas two copies of *DMRT1* are necessary. Furthermore, artificial dosage compensation (the experimental knock down of *DMRT1* expression) in ZZ embryos results in the feminization of developing gonads.

27. In snapping turtles, sex determination is strongly influenced by temperature such that males are favored in the 26–34°C range. Lizards, on the other hand, appear to have their sex determined by factors other than temperature in the 20–40°C range.

Chapter 6: Chromosome Mutations: Variation in Number and Arrangement

Concept Areas	Corresponding Problems
Variation in Chromosome Number	1, 2, 3, 4, 5, 6, 7, 8, 13, 14, 15, 16, 17, 18, 22, 23, 24, 25, 26
Nondisjunction	1, 3, 5, 18, 23, 25
Deletions	2, 9
Duplications	1, 2, 9, 12
Inversions	2, 3, 10, 11, 19, 27
Translocations	2, 20, 21, 22, 24, 26

Structures and Processes Checklist—Significant items that deserve special attention are identified with a "*".

(Check topic when mastered–provide examples where appropriate–understand the context of each entry)

- **Overview**
  - chromosome mutations*
  - chromosome aberrations
- **Variation in Chromosome Number***
  - aneuploidy*
  - euploidy*
  - polyploidy*
  - triploid
  - tetraploid
  - Klinefelter syndrome
  - Turner syndrome
  - nondisjunction*
- **Monosomy and Trisomy**
  - monosomy $(2n - 1)$*
  - haploinsufficiency
  - trisomy $(2n + 1)$*
  - Down syndrome
- trisomy 21 (47, 21+)
- Down syndrome critical region (DSCR)
- *DSCR1* gene
- nondisjunction, mostly in meiosis I*
- maternal age*
- amniocentesis
- chorionic villus sampling (CVS)
- noninvasive prenatal genetic diagnosis (NIPGD)
- Patau syndrome (47, 13+)
- Edwards syndrome (47, 18+)
- **Polyploidy in Plants**
  - autopolyploidy*
  - allopolyploidy*
  - autotriploids*
  - autotetraploids*

- commercial applications
- G1 cyclins*
- cell size increase
- allotetraploids*
- amphidiploids*
- **Variations in Composition** *
  - chromosome breakage
  - loss of segments
  - gain of segments
  - rearrangement of segments
  - aberration heterozygote*
- **Missing Regions**
  - deletion, or deficiency*
  - terminal deletion
  - intercalary deletion
  - deletion, or compensation, loop*
  - cri du chat syndrome (46,5p–)
  - partial monosomy
  - segmental deletion
  - *telomerase reverse transcriptase (TERT) gene*
- **Repeated Segments**
  - duplication*
  - rDNA
  - gene redundancy
  - gene amplification
  - nucleolar organizer region (NOR)
  - *Bar* mutation in *Drosophila*
  - gene duplications in evolution*
  - multigene families*
  - copy number variation (CNV)*

- positive and negative associations with human disease
- **Rearranged Gene Sequences**
  - inversion*
  - breakage and reinsertion
  - paracentric inversion*
  - pericentric inversion*
  - inversion heterozygotes*
  - inversion loop*
  - dicentric chromatid
  - acentric chromatid
  - dicentric bridges
  - suppressed recovery of crossover products*
  - evolutionary advantages*
  - balancer chromosomes
- **Altered Location in Genome**
  - translocation*
  - reciprocal translocation
  - unorthodox synapsis
  - semisterility*
  - Robertsonian translocation
  - familial Down syndrome*
  - balanced translocation
- **Sites Susceptible to Breakage**
  - fragile sites*
  - fragile-X syndrome (FXS)
  - *FMR1* gene
  - trinucleotide repeats*
  - genetic anticipation*
  - fragile sites and cancer

F6.1 Illustration of the chromosomal configurations of euploid and aneuploid genomes of *Drosophila melanogaster*.

Drosophila melanogaster female

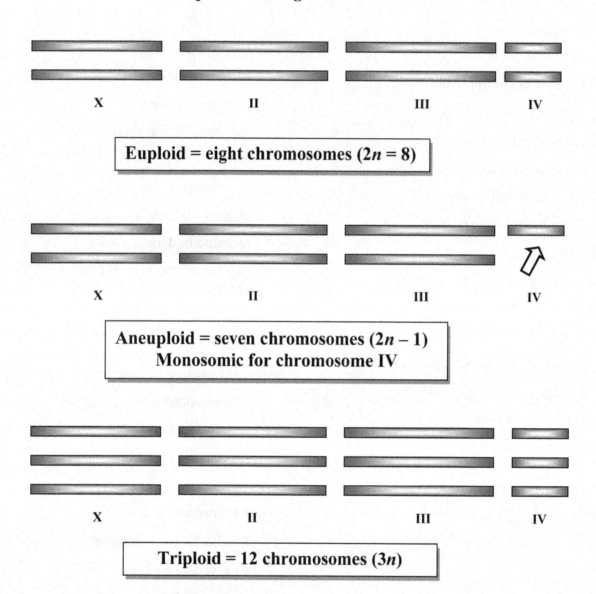

66

Answers to Now Solve This

6.1 The woman with Turner syndrome (sex chromosome composition of XO) could have inherited her sole X chromosome from either her father or her mother. Because both she and her father express hemophilia, it is likely that she inherited the X chromosome from the father and no sex chromosome from her mother. This means that nondisjunction occurred in the mother, either during meiosis I or meiosis II, producing an egg with no X chromosome. See text Figure 6.1 for a diagram of nondisjunction during the first and second meiotic divisions.

6.2 Interspecific hybrid might have an odd number of chromosomes or no/partial homology between the parental chromosomes. Either would cause a high proportion of univalents in meiosis I, resulting in the observed sterility. As such, viable gametes are rare and the likelihood of two such gametes "meeting" is remote. The horticulturist might attempt to reverse the sterility by treating the hybrid with colchicine, which, if successful, would double the chromosome number, so each chromosome would have a homolog with which to pair during meiosis.

6.3 Rare double crossovers *within the boundaries* of a paracentric inversion heterozygote produce only minor departures from the standard chromosomal arrangement as long as the crossovers involve the same two chromatids. With two-strand double crossovers, the second crossover negates the first. However, three-strand and four-strand double crossovers have consequences that lead to anaphase bridges as well as a high degree of genetically unbalanced gametes.

Chapter 6 Chromosome Mutations: Variation in Number and Arrangement

Solutions to Problems and Discussion Questions

1.

(a) Before the advent of polymorphic markers, maternal involvement in trisomy 21 was strongly suspected because of the striking influence of maternal age on incidence.

(b) Karyotype analysis of spontaneously aborted fetuses has shown that a significant percentage are trisomic and that any of the chromosomes can be involved. Other forms of aneuploidy (monosomy, nullisomy) are less represented.

(c) Studies in plants and animals have linked specific chromosomal changes with specific consistent phenotypes. For example, in jimson weed, each of the 12 possible trisomic conditions produces a unique alteration of the plant's capsule.

(d) By examining the polytene chromosomes of *Drosophila*, Bridges and Muller determined that the *Bar*-eye phenotype was caused by a chromosomal duplication of the 16A region on the X chromosome. In addition, unequal crossing over that resulted in reduced or increased numbers of 16A regions reverted or enhanced the *Bar*-eye phenotype.

2. Your essay can draw from information presented in the text that provides examples of deletions, duplications, inversions, translocations, and copy number variations.

3. With exceptions (mostly in plants) organisms typically inherit one chromosome complement (a haploid set (n) with one representative of each chromosome) from each parent. Such organisms are diploid, or $2n$. When an organism contains complete multiples of the n complement ($2n$, $3n$, $4n$, $5n$, etc.), it is said to be *euploid*, in contrast with *aneuploid*, in which complete haploid sets do not occur. An example of an aneuploid is trisomy, where a single chromosome is added to the $2n$ complement. In humans, trisomy 21 would be symbolized as $2n + 1$ or 47, 21+.

Monosomy is an aneuploid condition in which one member of a chromosome pair is missing, thus producing the chromosomal formula of $2n - 1$. Turner syndrome is an example of monosomy in humans. *Trisomy* is the chromosomal condition of $2n + 1$, whereby an extra chromosome is present. Down syndrome is an example in humans (47, 21+). Refer to the karyotype in text Figure 6.2: Notice that all the chromosomes are present in the diploid state except chromosome 21.

Patau syndrome is a chromosomal condition in which there is an extra D group chromosome. Such individuals are 47, 13+ and have multiple congenital malformations. *Edwards syndrome* is a chromosomal condition in which there is an extra E group chromosome (47, 18+). Individuals with Edwards syndrome have multiple congenital malformations and reduced life expectancy.

Polyploidy refers to instances in which there are more than two haploid sets of chromosomes in an individual cell. *Autopolyploidy* refers to cases of polyploidy in which the chromosomes originate from the same species. *Allopolyploidy* involves instances in which the chromosomes originate from the hybridization of two different species, usually closely related.

Autotetraploids arise within a species, whereas *amphidiploids* arise from two taxa followed by chromosome doubling.

Pericentric inversions are those that include the centromere in the inverted segment, whereas *paracentric* inversions do not include the centromere.

4. haploid = 9
triploid = 27
tetraploid = 36
trisomic = 19
monosomic = 17

5. Primary oocytes are formed by birth in females, and it isn't until just before ovulation that meiosis I is completed and at fertilization that meiosis II is completed. Because progression of meiosis is not continuous, it has been suggested that the long period of chromosomal synapsis and recombination may be involved in the nondisjunctional process in females.

6. An allotetraploid is created by fertilization between different species, followed by a doubling of chromosomes. Therefore, allotetraploids will be able to produce bivalents in meiosis I. In autotetraploids, each additional set of chromosomes is identical to the parent species. With four copies of similar chromosomes, an autotetraploid would also form bivalents in meiosis I. The fertility of these two types of polyploid individuals is probably equivalent. Both would be more fertile than autotriploids, which have an odd number of chromosomes and would frequently produce unbalanced gametes.

7. Two explanations were presented in the text. The first suggests that, due to the absence of a homologous chromosome, lethal alleles that were previously masked by their wild-type counterparts are now expressed. The second explanation is that monosomy can result in insufficient levels of certain required gene products, leading to death.

8. Cultivated American cotton has 26 pairs of chromosomes: 13 large, 13 small. Old World cotton has 13 pairs of large chromosomes, and wild American cotton has 13 pairs of small chromosomes. It is likely that an interspecific hybridization occurred followed by chromosome doubling. These events probably produced a fertile amphidiploid. Experiments have been conducted that appear to reconstruct the origin of cultivated American cotton.

9. Basically, the synaptic configurations produced by chromosomes bearing a deletion or duplication (on one homolog) are very similar. There will be point-for-point pairing in all sections that are capable of pairing. The section that has no homolog will "loop out," as shown in text Figure 6.10.

10. Although there is the appearance that crossing over is suppressed in inversion heterozygotes, the phenomenon extends from the fact that the crossover chromatids end up being abnormal in genetic content. As such, they fail to produce viable (or competitive) gametes or lead to zygotic or embryonic death. Notice in the text that the crossover chromatids end up genetically unbalanced. Therefore, rather than suppressing crossing over, the inversion actually suppresses the recovery of crossover products.

11. The best way to approach this problem is to draw out the chromosomes and the resulting crossover products. Crossing over in the inversion loop of a pericentric heterozygote produces all chromatids with centromeres, but the two chromatids involved in the crossover are genetically unbalanced. The balanced chromatids are of normal or inverted sequence.

12. Modern globin genes resulted from a duplication event in an ancestral gene about 500 million years ago. Mutations occurred over time, and a chromosomal aberration separated the duplicated genes, leaving the eventual α cluster on chromosome 16 and the eventual β cluster on chromosome 11. In a work entitled *Evolution by Gene Duplication*, Ohno suggests that gene duplication has been essential in the origin of new genes. If gene products serve essential functions, then mutation, and therefore evolution, would not be possible unless these gene products could be compensated by products of duplicated, normal genes. The duplicated genes, or the original genes themselves, would be able to undergo mutational "experimentation" without necessarily threatening the survival of the organism.

13. The primrose, *Primula kewensis*, with its 36 chromosomes, is likely to have formed from the hybridization and subsequent chromosome doubling of a cross between the two other species, each with 18 chromosomes.

14. Given the basic haploid complement of nine unique chromosomes, other forms with "*n* multiples" are said to be euploid, diploid (for 2*n*), or polyploid (for multiples above 2), and all are autoploid. Karyotypes would share the same basic chromosome set, with the appropriate number of copies of each chromosome (for example, four copies of each in an autotetraploid, as in the following illustration).

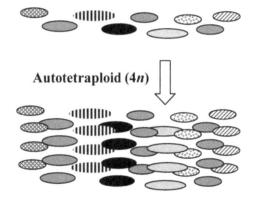

Basic set of nine unique chromosomes (*n*)

Autotetraploid (4*n*)

Individuals with 27 chromosomes are triploids (3*n*) and likely to be sterile because there are trivalents at meiosis I, which cause a relatively high number of unbalanced gametes to be formed.

15. Set up the cross in the usual manner, realizing that recessive genes in the monosomic IV individual will be expressed.

Let b = bent bristles; b^+ = normal bristles.

The underscore symbol (_) indicates a missing homolog.

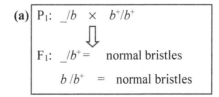

(a) P₁: _/b   × b^+/b^+

F₁: _/b^+ =   normal bristles

        b/b^+ =   normal bristles

Because the *bent* gene is autosomal, the two F_1 genotypes shown previously can occur in both males and females. In the text, monosomic IV flies were described as showing reduced body size. Assuming one can distinguish diploid from monosomic flies by size, the following $F_1 \times F_1$ cross can be performed:

F_2: _/b^+ ⇧ b/b^+

_/b^+	=	normal bristles
_/b	=	bent bristles
b^+/b^+	=	normal bristles
b/b^+	=	normal bristles

In this cross, only monosomic F_2 flies will have bent bristles.

(b) P_1: _/b^+ × b/b

⇩

F_1: _/b = bent bristles

b/b^+ = normal bristles

F_2: _/b × b/b^+

⇩

_/b^+	=	normal bristles
_/b	=	bent bristles
b^+/b	=	normal bristles
b/b	=	bent bristles

In this cross, bent bristles would be observed in both monosomic and diploid flies.

16. The cross would be as follows:

WWWW × *wwww*

F_1: *WWww*   all will have green seeds

F_2:   1*WW*   4*Ww*   1*ww*

1*WW*	
4*Ww*	35 *W – – –* and 1 *wwww*
1*ww*	

Thirty-five will have green seeds, since only a single dominant allele is needed to produce green seeds, and only one, the fully recessive genotype (*wwww*), will have white seeds.

17. Given some of the information in the preceding problem, the expression would be as follows:

(35/36 *W – – –* :1/36 *wwww*) ×
(35/36 *A – – –* :1/36 *aaaa*) ⟱

(35/36)(35/36)   *W – – – A – – –*

(35/36)(1/36)   *W – – – aaaa*

(35/36)(1/36)   *wwww A – – –*

(1/36)(1/36)   *wwwwaaaa*

18. Because two Gl_1 alleles and two ws_3 alleles are present in the triploid, they must have come from the pollen parent. The wording of the problem implies that the pollen parent contributed an unreduced (2*n*) gamete; however, another explanation, dispermic fertilization, is possible. In this case, two Gl_1ws_3 gametes could have fertilized the ovule.

19. (a) Chromosome 1 is metacentric. An inversion covering 70 percent of its length would produce a pericentric inversion. In all probability, crossing over in the inversion loop during spermatogenesis produced defective, unbalanced chromatids, thus leading to stillbirths and/or malformed children.

(b) It is probable that a significant proportion (perhaps 50 percent if there is a high frequency of crossing over in the inversion) of the man's children will be similarly influenced by the inversion.

(c) Because the karyotypic abnormality is observable, it may be possible to detect some of the abnormal chromosomes of the fetus by amniocentesis, CVS, or NIPDG. However, depending on the frequency and extent of crossover and the ability to detect minor changes in banding patterns, not all abnormal chromosomes may be detected.

20. (a) reciprocal translocation

(b)

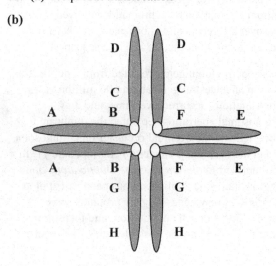

(c) No, this is not surprising because all chromosomal segments are present and there is no apparent loss of chromosomal material. If, however, the breakpoints for the translocation occurred within genes, then an abnormal phenotype might have resulted. In addition, a gene's function is sometimes influenced by its position—its neighboring genes, in other words. If such "position effects" occur, then a different phenotype might have resulted.

21.

(a) It is likely that the translocation described previously is the cause of the miscarriages. Segregation of the chromosomal elements will produce approximately half unbalanced gametes, giving her a 50 percent chance of having an affected child.

(b) Whether or not she should abandon her attempts to have a child is more a personal choice question than a science question. It is the task of the scientific community to provide accurate information within the limits of technology. Generally speaking, this information is provided to individuals so that they can make informed decisions.

(c) There is a 50 percent chance that the woman could have a normal child; however, although phenotypically normal, there is a 50 percent chance that a normal child will be a translocation carrier.

22. The symbol t(14;21) indicates that part of chromosome 21 is translocated to chromosome 14. When a gamete with a t(14;21) chromosome and a normal chromosome 21 combines with a standard haploid gamete during fertilization, the resulting zygote has 46 chromosomes, but effectively has three copies of chromosome 21.

23. (a) The father, who has both the X-linked skin condition and a Y chromosome, must have contributed the abnormal gamete to produce a male child who is also heterozygous for anhidrotic dysplasia.

(b) Nondisjunction must have occurred during meiosis I of spermatogenesis.

(c) This son's phenotype is a mosaic of normal and abnormal skin. This pattern is the result of the random inactivation of one of his two X chromosomes (a form of dosage compensation) in each of his cells.

24. First consider what is meant by a Robertsonian translocation: Breaks occur at the short arms of two nonhomologous acrocentric chromosomes. The small acentric fragments are lost, and the larger chromosomal segments fuse at or near the centromeric region. This produces a compound, larger submetacentric or metacentric chromosome. Following is a description of breakage/reunion events that illustrate such a translocation in the relatively small, similarly sized chromosomes 19 (metacentric) and 20 (metacentric/submetacentric). The case described here is shown occurring before S phase duplication. The parents were each heterozygous for the translocation; that is, they each have one normal chromosome 19, one normal chromosome 20, and one Robertsonian t(19;20). This is the only way they could produce both "homozygous" and "heterozygous" children. Stillbirths might have resulted from genetically unbalanced gametes caused by various segregation products of meiosis. Because the likelihood of such a translocation is fairly small in a general population, inbreeding played a significant role in allowing the translocation to "meet itself."

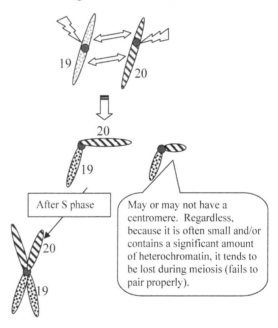

25. It is likely that mitotic nondisjunction contributed to the mosaic condition. If one of the X chromosomes failed to be included in a daughter mitotic cleavage cell, then a substantial proportion of the child's cells would be XO. Expression of Turner syndrome characteristics would depend on the percentage and location of the XO cell population.

26. This female will produce meiotic products of the following six possible types:

normal: 18 + 21
translocated: 18/21
translocated plus 21: 18/21 + 21
deficient for 21: 18 only
translocated plus 18: 18/21 + 18
deficient for18: 21 only

As noted in the textbook, the latter two possibilities are rare.

Fertilization with a normal 18 + 21 sperm cell will produce the following offspring (father's contribution in boldface):

normal: 46 chromosomes
translocation carrier: 45 chromosomes 18/21 + **18 + 21**
trisomy 21: 46 chromosomes 18/21 + 21 + **21 + 18**
monosomic for 21: 45 chromosomes 18 + **18 + 21** (lethal)
trisomy 18: 46 chromosomes 18/21 +18 +**18 + 21**
monosomic for 18: 21 + **21 + 18** (lethal)

27. Considering that there are at least three map units between each of the loci and that only four phenotypes are observed, it is likely that genes *a b c d* are included in an inversion, and crossovers that do occur among these genes are not recovered because of their genetically unbalanced nature. In a sense, the minimum distance between loci *d* and *e* can be estimated as 10 map units:

$$(48 + 52/1000)$$

However, this is actually the distance from the *e* locus to the breakpoint that includes the inversion.

The "map" is therefore as drawn below:

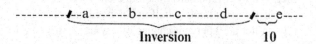

Chapter 7: Linkage and Chromosome Mapping in Eukaryotes

Concept Areas	Corresponding Problems
Linkage vs. Independent Assortment	1, 2, 10, 15, 16, 21
Gene Mapping	1, 8, 9, 10, 11, 12, 14, 15, 17, 18, 19, 20, 21, 22, 24
Multiple Crossovers	4, 6, 7, 13, 14, 18
Determining Gene Sequence	9, 14, 20
Interference and Coefficient of Coincidence	7, 14
Crossing Over in the Four-Strand Stage	1, 3, 5, 18
Mechanism of Crossing Over	1, 2, 3, 4, 5, 6, 23, 25
Human Maps	24

Structures and Processes Checklist—Significant items that deserve special attention are identified with a "*".

(Check topic when mastered–provide examples where appropriate–understand the context of each entry)

- o **Overview**
  - o linkage*
  - o crossing over
  - o recombination*
- o **Linked Genes Segregate Together**
  - o independent assortment*
  - o linkage without crossing over*
  - o linkage with crossing over*
  - o parental, or noncrossover, gametes*
  - o recombinant, or crossover, gametes*
  - o 50 percent maximum*
  - o linkage ratio
  - o horizontal line designation
  - o 1:2:1
  - o linkage group*

- o **Gene Mapping***
  - o Morgan, Sturtevant
  - o two X-linked genes
  - o chiasma (pl. chiasmata)
  - o points of genetic exchange
  - o linear order of linked genes
  - o crossing over
  - o frequencies are additive
  - o chromosome map*
  - o 1 map unit (mu) = 1 percent recombination
  - o autosomal linkage
  - o chromosome theory of inheritance
  - o single crossover*
  - o % recombinant tetrads = 2 × (percent recombinant gametes)*

Chapter 7 Linkage and Chromosome Mapping in Eukaryotes

- **Determining Gene Sequence***
  - multiple crossovers
  - double crossovers (DCOs)*
  - product law*
  - three-point mapping*
  - three criteria for mapping cross*
  - heterozygosity at all loci
  - progeny phenotypes reflect gamete genotypes
  - adequate progeny sample size
  - reciprocal classes*
  - noncrossovers (NCOs) = largest proportion of offspring*
  - DCOs = least frequent*

- **Mapping Accuracy***
  - undetected crossovers
  - multiple-strand exchanges
  - degree of inaccuracy depends on distance*
  - expected frequency of double crossovers (DCO$_{exp}$)
  - interference (*I*)
  - coefficient of coincidence (*C*)
  - $C = DCO_{obs} / DCO_{exp}$
  - $I = 1 - C$
  - positive interference
  - negative interference

- **Chromosome Mapping and Computers***
  - DNA markers*
  - useful landmarks
  - restriction fragment length polymorphisms (RFLPs)*
  - microsatellites*
  - single nucleotide polymorphisms (SNPs)
  - cystic fibrosis
  - sequence maps
  - bioinformatics
  - physical map vs. genetic map

- **Genetic Exchange**
  - physical exchange between chromatids
  - Creighton and McClintock
  - exchange during mitosis
  - sister chromatid exchanges (SCEs)*
  - bromodeoxyuridine (BrdU)
  - harlequin chromosomes
  - Bloom syndrome
  - *BLM* gene
  - DNA helicase

F7.1 Illustration of critical arrangements of linked genes. Notice that there are two possible arrangements for an *AaBb* double heterozygote. In order to do linkage problems correctly, such arrangements must be understood.

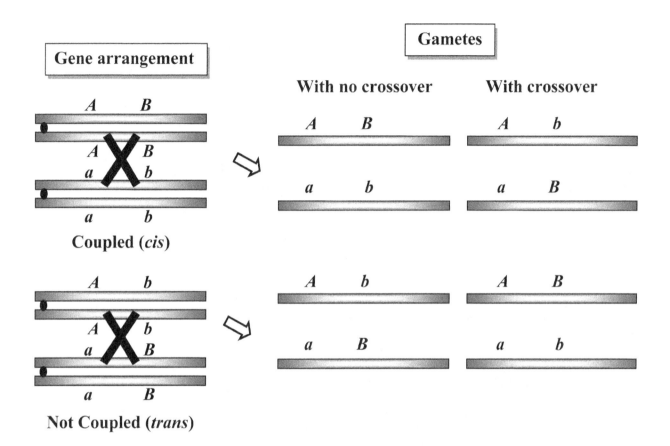

Answers to Now Solve This

7.1 The initial cross for this problem would be

AaBb × *aabb*

(a) If the two loci are on different chromosomes, independent assortment would occur, and the following distribution (1:1:1:1) is expected:

1/4   *AaBb*
1/4   *Aabb*
1/4   *aaBb*
1/4   *aabb*

(b) Even though the two loci are linked and on the same chromosome, the frequency of crossing over is so high that crossovers always occur. Under that condition, independent assortment would occur, and the following distribution (1:1:1:1) is expected:

1/4   *AaBb*
1/4   *Aabb*
1/4   *aaBb*
1/4   *aabb*

(c) If crossovers never occur, then all of the gametes from the heterozygous parent are *parental,* and a 1:1 distribution is expected. If the arrangement is

AB/*ab* × *ab*/*ab*

then the two types of offspring will be as follows:

1/2   *AB*/*ab*
1/2   *ab*/*ab*

Under this condition, *AB* are *coupled* (Also see F7.1). If, however, *A* and *B* are not coupled, then the symbolism would be

Ab/*aB* × *aabb*

The offspring would occur as follows:

1/2   *Ab*/*ab*
1/2   *aB*/*ab*

7.2 Because there is no indication as to the configuration of the *P* and *Z* genes (*coupled or not coupled*) in the parent, one must look at the percentages in the offspring. Notice that the most frequent classes are *PZ* and *pz*. These classes represent the parental (noncrossover) groups, which indicates that the original parental arrangement in the testcross was

PZ/*pz* × *pz*/*pz*

Adding the crossover percentages together (6.9 + 7.1) gives 14 percent, so the map distance between the two genes is 14 map units (14 mu).

7.3 In typical trihybrid crosses, one expects eight kinds of offspring. In this example, only six are listed; because the double crossover class is the least frequent, one can assume that it is this class that is not represented.

To work this type of problem, examine the data to see which genotypes are not present. In this case, the double crossover class consists of the following:

<u>+ + c</u>   and   <u>a b +</u>

(a) Compare the parental classes (most frequent) with the double crossover classes (zero in this case), and use the method described in the text to determine that the gene *b* is in the middle and the arrangement is as follows:

<u>+ b c</u>   (This can also be written as + *b c/ a* + +.)
a + +

(b) Calculate the distance between genes by adding the numbers of single and double crossover, dividing by the total number of progeny, and finally multiplying by 100 (to determine percentage). Note: For consistency, the zeros (double crossovers) are included in the calculations.

$a - b$ $\quad = \dfrac{32 + 38 + 0 + 0}{1000} \times 100$

$\qquad = 7$ map units

$b - c$ $\quad = \dfrac{11 + 9 + 0 + 0}{1000} \times 100$

$\qquad = 2$ map units

The map would appear as follows:

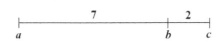

(c) The progeny phenotypes that are missing are + + *c* and *a b* +. In a population of 1000 offspring, (0.07 × 0.02 × 1000) = 1.4 (or 0.7 each) would be expected. It is likely that the sample size was too small to reliably detect such infrequently occurring genotypes.

Solutions to Problems and Discussion Questions

1. (a) Morgan and his students, especially Alfred Sturtevant, correlated chiasma frequency with the distance between linked genes. Genes that were farther apart exhibited more frequent chiasmata and, therefore, more frequent crossovers. The most important hint was that recombination frequency between genes *a* and *c* could be equal to recombination frequency between *a* and *b* plus recombination frequency between *b* and *c*.

(b) The discovery that genes segregated together during gamete formation indicated a physical association among genes.

(c) Two experimental lines, one using maize (Creighton and McClintock) and the other using *Drosophila*, showed that each time a crossover occurred, an actual physical exchange between chromosomes also occurred. Each experiment demonstrated a switch in cytological chromosomal markers when genetic markers exchanged.

(d) Even though exchanges between sister chromatids do not produce new allelic combinations, they can be demonstrated using molecular markers such as bromodeoxyuridine.

2. Your essay should include methods of detection through crosses with appropriate, distinguishable markers, as well as the fact that, in most cases, the frequency of crossing over is directly related to the distance between genes.

3. First, in order for chromosomes to engage in crossing over, they must be in proximity. It is likely that the side-by-side pairing that occurs during synapsis is the earliest time during the cell cycle that chromosomes achieve that necessary proximity. Second, chiasmata are visible during prophase I of meiosis, and it is likely that these structures are intimately associated with the genetic event of crossing over.

4. With some qualification, especially around the centromeres and telomeres, one can say that crossing over is somewhat randomly distributed over the length of the chromosome. Two loci that are far apart are more likely to experience a random crossover event between them than are two loci that are close together.

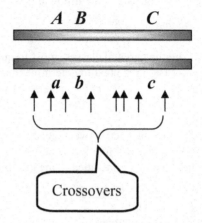

5. Crossing over occurs at the four-strand stage of the cell cycle (that is, after S phase), such that each single crossover involves only two (50 percent) of the four chromatids.

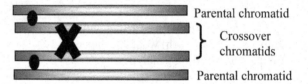

6. As mentioned in an earlier answer (Problem 4), with some qualifications, crossovers occur randomly along the lengths of chromosomes. Within any region, the occurrence of two events is less likely than the occurrence of one event. If the probability of one event is $1/X$, and the probability of a second event is $1/Y$, then the probability of two events occurring at the same time will be the product of the individual probabilities, or $1/(XY)$. This value will be smaller than either single probability.

7. Positive interference occurs when a crossover in one region of a chromosome interferes with crossovers in nearby regions. Such interference ranges from 0 (no interference) to 1.0 (complete interference). Interference is often explained by a physical rigidity of chromatids such that they are unlikely to make sufficiently sharp bends to allow crossovers to be close together.

8. One of the parents must be heterozygous at all loci being mapped. If crossover in an organism is limited to one sex, the heterozygous individual must be of the sex in which crossing over occurs. In other words, it would be useless to map genes in *Drosophila* if the male parent is the heterozygote, since crossing over is not typical in *Drosophila* males.

In addition, the cross must be set up so that the phenotypes of the offspring readily reveal their genotypes. The best arrangement is one in which a heterozygous individual is crossed with another that is fully recessive for the genes being mapped.

Finally, sufficient progeny must be generated to ensure observation of rare crossover products.

9. Because the distance between *dp* and *ap* is greatest when compared to the other distances, they must be on the "outside," and *cl* must be in the middle. The genetic map would be as follows:

$$dp\text{--- }cl\text{----------------------}ap$$

3 *mu*   39 *mu*

10. In looking at this problem, one can immediately conclude that the two loci (kernel color and plant color) are linked because the testcross progeny occur in a ratio other than 1:1:1:1 (and epistasis does not appear because all phenotypes expected are present). The question is whether the arrangement in the parents is *coupled* (See F7.1):

$$RY/ry \quad \times \quad ry/ry$$

or *not coupled*:

$$Ry/rY \quad \times \quad ry/ry$$

The most frequent phenotypes in the offspring (the noncrossover or parental phenotypes) are colored, green (88) and colorless, yellow (92). This indicates that the heterozygous parent in the testcross is coupled or *RY/ry*, with the two dominant alleles on one chromosome and the two recessives on the homolog. In addition, there are 20 crossover progeny among the 200, or 20/200. The map distance between the *R* and *Y* loci is, therefore, 10 map units (20/200 × 100 to convert to percentages).

11. Start this problem by working through the expected offspring under two models, one with no crossing over and the second with 30 percent crossing over in the female.

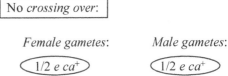

Female gametes: *Male gametes:*

1/2 *e ca⁺*   1/2 *e ca⁺*

1/2 *e⁺ ca*   1/2 *e⁺ ca*

Offspring:

    1/4   *e* phenotype

    2/4   wild

    1/4   *ca* phenotype

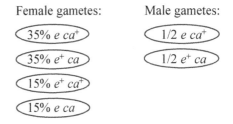

Female gametes: Male gametes:

35% *e ca⁺*   1/2 *e ca⁺*

35% *e⁺ ca*   1/2 *e⁺ ca*

15% *e⁺ ca⁺*

15% *e ca*

Offspring (obtained by combining gametes and phenotypes):

e phenotype = 17.5% + 7.5%   **= 25%**

wild phenotype =
   17.5% + 7.5% + 17.5% + 7.5% **= 50%**

ca phenotype = 17.5% + 7.5%   **= 25%**

Therefore, the distribution of phenotypes is the same, regardless of the contribution of the crossover classes.

12. This problem can be approached by looking for the most distant loci (*adp* and *b*) and then filling in the intermediate loci. In this case, the map for parts **(a)** and **(b)** is the following:

d.........	*b*..........	*pr*.........	*vg*........	*c*........	*adp*
31	48	54	67	75	83

Map units

The expected map units between *d* and *c* would be 44, between *d* and *vg* 36, and between *d* and *adp* 52. However, because there is a theoretical maximum of 50 percent recombination frequency possible between two loci in any one cross, the latter distance would be below the 52 determined by simple subtraction.

13.

	female A	female B	Frequency
NCO	3, 4	7, 8	first
SCO	1, 2	3, 4	second
SCO	7, 8	5, 6	third
DCO	5, 6	1, 2	fourth

The single crossover classes that represent crossovers between the genes that are closer together (*d–b*) would occur less frequently than the single crossover classes between more distant genes (*b–c*).

14. For two reasons, it is clear that the genes are in the *coupled* configuration in the F_1 female. First, a completely homozygous female was mated to a wild-type male, and second, the phenotypes of the offspring indicate the following parental classes

$$sc \; s \; v \text{ and } + + +$$

(a)

$P_1: sc \; s \; v \, / sc \; s \; v \quad \times \quad + + + / Y$

$F_1: + + + / sc \; s \; v \quad \times \quad sc \; s \; v / Y$

(b) Examine the parental classes (most frequent) and compare the arrangement with the double crossover classes (least frequent). Notice that the *v* gene "switches places" between the two groups (parentals and double crossovers). The gene that switches places is in the middle.

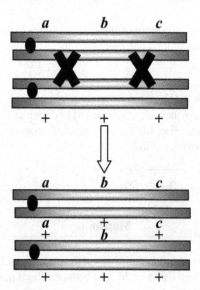

The map distances are determined by first writing the proper arrangement and sequence of genes, and then computing the distances between each set of genes.

$$\frac{sc \; v \; s}{+ + +}$$

$$sc - v = \frac{150 + 156 + 10 + 14}{1000} \times 100$$

$$= 33 \text{ percent (map units)}$$

$$v - s = \frac{46 + 30 + 10 + 14}{1000} \times 100$$

$$= 10 \text{ percent (map units)}$$

Double crossovers are always added into each crossover group because they represent a crossover in each region.

$$\underset{33}{sc\text{-------}}\underset{10}{v\text{-----}s}$$

(c) The expected number of double crossovers is calculated by multiplying the frequencies of each single crossover and then multiplying by the total population size. Therefore, $DCO_{exp} = (0.33 \times 0.1) \times 1000 = 33$. Because only 24 double-crossover individuals were observed, there were fewer than expected.

(d) The coefficient of coincidence = C

$$C = \frac{\text{observed freq. double C/O}}{\text{expected freq. double C/O}}$$

$$= \frac{(14 + 10)/1000}{0.33 \times 0.1}$$

$$= \frac{0.024}{0.033} = 0.727$$

Interference is given by I, where $I = 1 - C$. In this case, $I = 1 - 0.727 = 0.273$. Because this is a positive number, it indicates that positive chromosomal interference is present.

15. (a) There are several ways to think through this problem. Remember that there is no crossing over in *Drosophila* males. Therefore, any gene on the same chromosome will be completely linked to any other gene on the same chromosome. Because you can get *pink* by itself, *short* cannot be completely linked to this gene. This leaves linkage to *black* on chromosome II, or a locus on either chromosome IV, or the X chromosome. Because the distribution of phenotypes in males and females is essentially the same, the gene cannot be X-linked. In addition, the F_1 males were wild, and if the *short* gene were on the X, the F_1 males would be short.

It is also reasonable to state that the gene cannot be on chromosome IV because there would be eight phenotypic classes (independent assortment of three genes) instead of the four observed. Through these insights, one can conclude that the *short* gene is on chromosome II with the *black* gene.

Another way to approach this type of problem is to make three chromosomal configurations possible in the F_1 male. By producing gametes from this male, the answer becomes obvious.

Case A	Case B	Case C
p b *sh*	*p sh* *b*	*b sh* *p*
+ + +	+ + +	+ + +

Develop the gametes from case C and cross them out to the completely recessive triple mutant. You will get the results in the table.

(b) The testcross is now the following:

> Females: $\dfrac{b\,sh}{+\,+}\quad \dfrac{p}{+}$ × Males: $\dfrac{b\,sh}{b\,sh}\quad \dfrac{p}{p}$

The new gametes, which result from crossing over in the female, would be *b +* and *+ sh*. Because the gene *p* is assorting independently, it is not important in this discussion. Because 15 percent of the offspring now contain these recombinant chromatids, the map distance between the *black* and *short* must be 15 mu.

16. Because two of the genes are linked and 20 map units apart on chromosome III, and one is on chromosome II, the problem is a combination of linkage and independent assortment. First, provide the genotypes of the parents in the original cross and the reciprocal. Use a semicolon to indicate that two different chromosome pairs are involved.

> P_1:
>
> females: $+/+$; $p\,e/p\,e$
>
> ×
>
> males: dp/dp; $+ +/+ +$
>
> F_1: $+/dp$; $+ +/p\,e$

> Testcross
>
> females: $+/dp$; $+ +/p\,e$
>
> ×
>
> males: dp/dp; $p\,e/p\,e$

Female gametes: Use a modification of the forked-line method for determining the types of gametes to be produced. The *dumpy* locus will give $0.5 +$ and $0.5\ dp$ to the gametes because of independent assortment (on a different chromosome), and the other two loci will segregate with 20 percent being the recombinants and 80 percent being the parentals.

$$0.5 + \begin{cases} 0.4 + & + \text{ (parental)} & = 0.20 + + + \\ 0.1 + & e \text{ (crossover)} & = 0.05 + + e \\ 0.1\ p & + \text{ (crossover)} & = 0.05 + p + \\ 0.4\ p & e \text{ (parental)} & = 0.20 + p\ e \end{cases}$$

$$0.5\ dp \begin{cases} 0.4 + & + \text{ (parental)} & = 0.20\ dp + + \\ 0.1 + & e \text{ (crossover)} & = 0.05\ dp + e \\ 0.1\ p & + \text{ (crossover)} & = 0.05\ dp\ p + \\ 0.4\ p & e \text{ (parental)} & = 0.20\ dp\ p\ e \end{cases}$$

Crossed with *dp p e* from the male gives the following offspring:

> 0.20 wild type
> 0.05 ebony
> 0.05 pink
> 0.20 pink, ebony
> 0.20 dumpy
> 0.05 dumpy, ebony
> 0.05 dumpy, pink
> 0.20 dumpy, pink, ebony

For the reciprocal cross,

> Testcross
>
> males: $+/dp$; $+ +/p\,e$
>
> ×
>
> females: dp/dp; $p\,e/p\,e$

there would be no crossover classes.

$$0.5 + \begin{cases} 0.5 + & + \text{ (parental)} = 0.25 + + + \\ 0.5\ p & e \text{ (parental)} = 0.25 + p\ e \end{cases}$$

$$0.5\ dp \begin{cases} 0.5 + & + \text{ (parental)} = 0.25\ dp + + \\ 0.5\ p & e \text{ (parental)} = 0.25\ dp\ p\ e \end{cases}$$

Crossing with *dp p e* from the female gives the following offspring:

> 0.25 wild type
> 0.25 pink, ebony
> 0.25 dumpy
> 0.25 dumpy, pink, ebony

The results would change because of the absence of crossing over in males.

17. Because *Stubble* is a dominant mutation and *curled* is a recessive mutation, one would use the typical testcross arrangement with males homozygous for recessive alleles at both loci. Therefore, the arrangement would be

  + *cu*/ + *cu*

18. First, make a drawing with the genes placed on the homologous chromosomes as follows:

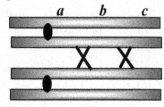

Realize that there are four chromatids in each tetrad and that a single crossover involves only two of the four chromatids. Noninvolved chromatids must be added to the noncrossover classes. Do all the crossover classes first, then add up the noncrossover chromatids. For example, in the first crossover class (20 between *a* and *b*), notice that there will be 40 chromatids that were not involved in the crossover. These 40 must be added to the *abc* and +++ classes.

a b c	=	168
+ + +	=	168
a + +	=	20
+ *b c*	=	20
+ + *c*	=	10
a b +	=	10
+ *b* +	=	2
a + *c*	=	2

Detailed explanation:
Sixty-eight of 100 tetrads show no crossover; therefore, 68 x 4 = 272 chromatids that are nonrecombinant. These are split equally between *abc* and +++, so we start at 136 each.

Twenty of 100 tetrads show crossover between *a* and *b*. This means that 20 x 2 = 40 chromatids are recombinant—these are split between *a*++ and +*bc*, so 20 each. There are also 40 chromatids that are not involved in crossover. These are added to the already accounted nonrecombinant chromatids with 20 being added to each genotype. This gives us 136 + 20 = 156 nonrecombinant chromatids each for *abc* and +++.

Ten of 100 tetrads show crossover between *b* and *c*. This means that 10 x 2 = 20 chromatids are recombinant—these are split between ++*c* and *ab*+, so 10 each. There are also 20 chromatids that are not involved in crossover. These are added to the already

accounted nonrecombinant chromatids with 10 being added to each genotype. So now we have 156 + 10 = 166 nonrecombinant chromatids each for *abc* and +++.

Finally, 2 of 100 tetrads show crossover between both *a* and *b* as well as *b* and *c*. This means that 2 x 2 = 4 chromatids are recombinant—these are split between +*b*+ and *a*+*c*, so 2 each. There are also 4 chromatids that are not involved in crossover. These are added to the already accounted nonrecombinant chromatids with 2 being added to each genotype. This gives us a final value of 166 + 2 = 168 nonrecombinant chromatids each for *abc* and +++.

The map distances would be computed as follows:

$$a - b = \frac{20 + 20 + 2 + 2}{400} \times 100$$
$$= 11 \text{ map units}$$

$$b - c = \frac{10 + 10 + 2 + 2}{400} \times 100$$
$$= 6 \text{ map units}$$

19. Assign the following symbols, for example:

  R = red   *r* = yellow
  O = oval   *o* = long

Genotype of parent plant A: *Ro/rO*
Genotype of parent plant B: *RO/ro*

The data indicate that the fruit color and fruit shape loci are on the same chromosome, separated by 10 map units.

20. (a) The cross will be as follows. Represent the *Dichaete* gene as an uppercase letter because it is dominant.

P₁:	*D* + +/ + + +	×	+ *e p*/+ *e p*
F₁:	*D* + +/+ *e p*	×	+ *e p*/+ *e p*
F₂:	*D* + +/+ *e p*	Dichaete	
	+ *e p*/+ *e p*	ebony, pink	
	D e +/+ *e p*	Dichaete, ebony	
	+ + *p*/+ *e p*	pink	
	D + *p*/+ *e p*	Dichaete, pink	
	+ *e* +/+ *e p*	ebony	
	D e p/+ *e p*	Dichaete, ebony, pink	
	+ + +/+ *e p*	wild type	

(b) Determine which gene is in the middle by comparing the parental classes with the double crossover classes. The *pink* gene is in the middle, so rewrite the sequence of genes with the correct arrangement, as follows:

$$F_1: \quad D + + / + p\, e \quad \times \quad + p\, e / + p\, e$$

Distances (remember to add in the double crossover classes):

$$D - p = \frac{12 + 13 + 2 + 3}{1000} \times 100$$
$$= 3.0 \text{ map units}$$

$$p - e = \frac{84 + 96 + 2 + 3}{1000} \times 100$$
$$= 18.5 \text{ map units}$$

21. (a) There would be $2^n = 8$ genotypic and phenotypic classes, and they would occur in a 1:1:1:1:1:1:1:1 ratio.

(b) There would be two classes, and they would occur in a 1:1 ratio.

(c) There are 20 map units between the A and B loci, and locus C assorts independently from both the A and B loci.

22. Genetic maps are more accurate when relatively small intergenic distances are covered and when large numbers of offspring are scored. Based on these criteria, the relative distance between the A and B genes might not be accurate. The map could be improved if recombination data for genes located between the A and B loci were included and if a larger sample size were used.

23. The purpose of the experiment was to determine whether genetic crossing over involved actual physical exchange of chromosomal material, a feature that was not required by other models of the time. By having microscopically visible markers on the chromosomes, Creighton and McClintock were able to show that homologous chromosomal material physically exchanged segments during crossing over.

24. DNA markers are unique DNA regions whose nucleotide sequence and chromosomal location are known and serve as landmarks for the mapping of genes. Typical markers include restriction fragment length polymorphisms (RFLPs), microsatellites, and single-nucleotide polymorphisms (SNPs). Because the number of DNA markers in an individual may be in the tens of thousands, they can "mark" small intervals of each of the 23 human chromosomes.

25. Because sister chromatids are genetically identical (with the exception of rare new mutations), crossing over between sisters provides no increase in genetic variability. Somatic crossing over would have no influence on the offspring produced.

Chapter 8: Genetic Analysis and Mapping in Bacteria and Bacteriophages

Concept Areas	Corresponding Problems
Genetic Recombination in Bacteria	1, 2, 3, 4, 5
Conjugation	1, 2, 3, 4, 5, 6, 7, 8
Transformation	1, 2, 3, 9
Bacteriophages	10, 11, 12, 13, 14, 15, 16, 17, 18, 19, 20
Transduction	1, 2, 3, 17, 18
Mapping	6, 18

Structures and Processes Checklist—Significant items that deserve special attention are identified with a "*".

(Check topic when mastered–provide examples where appropriate–understand the context of each entry)

- **Overview**
  - bacteria
  - bacteriophages
  - recombination*
  - chromosome mapping
- **Bacteria Mutate Spontaneously**
  - haploid
  - minimal medium*
  - prototroph*
  - auxotroph*
  - colony
  - serial dilution*
  - dilution factor*
- **Recombination in Bacteria**
  - genetic recombination*
  - replacement of gene(s)
  - vertical gene transfer*
  - horizontal gene transfer*

- conjugation*
- unidirectional transfer*
- F^+ cells*
- F^- cells*
- Davis U-tube
- physical contact required
- F pilus, or sex pilus (pl. pili)
- fertility factor (F factor)*
- rare genetic recombination
- transfer of F factor
- exconjugant
- Hfr, high-frequency recombination*
- Hfr recipients remain F^-
- nonrandom gene transfer
- interrupted mating*
- ordered transfer of genes*
- time mapping

- ○ point of origin (*O*)/origin of transfer*
- ○ F factor can carry bacterial genes
- ○ F' state*
- ○ merozygote
- ○ **F Factor and Plasmids***
  - ○ plasmid
  - ○ R plasmids*
  - ○ resistance transfer factor (RTF)
  - ○ r-determinants
  - ○ multiple antibiotic resistance*
  - ○ Col plasmid
  - ○ ColE1
  - ○ colicins
  - ○ colicinogenic
- ○ **Transformation and Recombination**
  - ○ transformation*
  - ○ extracellular DNA
  - ○ competence*
  - ○ complementary host region*
  - ○ heteroduplex
  - ○ cotransformation*
  - ○ linked genes
- ○ **Bacterial Viruses**
  - ○ bacteriophages, or phages*
- ○ bacteriophage T4
- ○ sequential assembly of virus
- ○ lysis*
- ○ lysozyme
- ○ plaque assay*
- ○ plaque
- ○ initial phage density = (plaque number/mL) × (dilution factor)
- ○ integration of DNA
- ○ lysogeny*
- ○ prophage*
- ○ temperate phages*
- ○ virulent phages*
- ○ lysogenic*
- ○ lytic
- ○ **Virus-Mediated Transfer**
  - ○ transduction*
  - ○ *Salmonella typhimurium*
  - ○ auxotrophic strains*
  - ○ filterable agent (FA)
  - ○ bacteriophage P22
  - ○ mapping*
  - ○ cotransduction*

Answers to Now Solve This

8.1 Approach this problem by lining up the data from the various crosses in the following order:

Hfr Strain		Order								
1	T	C	H	R	O					
2			H	R	O	M	B			
3		C	H	R	O	M	→			
4						M	B	A	K	T
5						B	A	K	T	C	→
Overall	T	C	H	R	O	M	B	A	K	

All of the genes can be linked to give a consistent map and with ends that overlap, indicating that the map is circular. The order of transfer is left-to-right, except for strains 3 and 5, where it is reversed (shown by →) due to integration of the F factor in the opposite orientation.

8.2 In the first dataset, the transformation of each locus, a^+ and b^+, occurs at a frequency of 0.031 and 0.012, respectively. To decide if there is linkage between a and b, determine whether the frequency of double transformants a^+b^+ is greater than that expected for two independent events. Multiplying 0.031×0.012 gives 0.00037, or approximately 0.04 percent—the same as the frequency reported. From this information, one would consider no linkage between these two loci. Notice that this frequency is approximately the same as the frequency reported in the second experiment, in which each locus is transformed independently.

Chapter 8 *Genetic Analysis and Mapping in Bacteria and Bacteriophages*

Solutions to Problems and Discussion Questions

1. (a) A variety of experiments involving transformation, conjugation, and transduction showed that genetic elements from one bacterial strain can be transferred to another strain. Historically, transformation set the stage for the discovery that DNA is the genetic material in bacteria.

(b) The general strategy for determining the dependence of cell-to-cell contact in one form of bacterial recombination involved a Davis U-tube and a filter. During conjugation, when the filter separated two auxotrophic strains, no genetic recombination occurred. We know that contact is the initial step by observation of the F pilus.

(c) Two auxotrophic strains were placed on opposite sides of a Davis U-tube apparatus. Although the filter eliminated the possibility of bacterial contact, a one-way passage of genetic material was detected. This filterable agent was insensitive to DNase treatment and was therefore not naked DNA.

2. Your essay should include a description of the following: conjugation, transformation, transduction in bacteria, whether recombination occurs and at what rate, and a summary of the consequences.

3. Three modes of recombination in bacteria are *conjugation, transformation,* and *transduction.* Conjugation is dependent on the F factor, which, by a variety of mechanisms, can direct genetic exchange between two bacterial cells. Transformation is the uptake of exogenous DNA by cells. Transduction is the exchange of genetic material using a bacteriophage as a carrier.

4. (a) The requirement for physical contact between bacterial cells during conjugation was established by placing a filter in a U-tube such that the medium can be exchanged but the bacteria cannot come in contact. Under this condition, conjugation does not occur.

(b) Early experiments suggested directionality, with one strain being the donor and the other being the recipient. Strains identified as donors could convert recipients into donors, but the converse was never true. Additional experimentation revealed that each donor strain contained a mobile fertility factor (the F factor). Further confirmation came from studies using Hfr bacteria.

(c) An F^+ bacterium contains a circular, double-stranded, structurally independent DNA molecule,

the F^+ factor plasmid, that can direct transfer of DNA from one cell to another.

5. In an $F^+ \times F^-$ cross, the transfer of the F factor converts a recipient bacterium from F^- to F^+. Any gene may be transferred, but the frequency of transfer is relatively low. Crosses that are Hfr $\times$ F^- produce recombinants at a higher frequency than the $F^+ \times F^-$ cross. The transfer is oriented (nonrandom) and the recipient cell usually remains F^-.

Bacteria that are F^+ possess the F factor and are the donors in conjugation, whereas those that are F^- lack the F factor and are conjugation recipients. In Hfr cells, the F factor is integrated into the bacterial chromosome, which allows the time-dependent, ordered transfer of bacterial genes into F^- recipients. F' bacteria arise from the imprecise excision of the F factor from an Hfr strain, such that the F factor carries bacterial genes that were adjacent to its insertion point in the bacterial chromosome. Any gene may be transferred on an F', and the frequency of transfer is relatively low.

6. Mapping the chromosome in an Hfr $\times$ F^- cross takes advantage of the oriented transfer of the bacterial chromosome through the conjugation tube. For each Hfr type, the point of insertion and the direction of transfer are fixed. Breaking the conjugation tube at different times produces exconjugants with correspondingly different lengths of the donor chromosome being transferred. Thus, mapping of genes is based on time.

7. In an Hfr $\times$ F^- cross, the F factor is directing the transfer of the donor chromosome. It takes approximately 100 minutes to transfer the entire bacterial chromosome. Because the F factor is the last element to be transferred and the conjugation tube is fragile, the likelihood for complete chromosomal transfer (including the F factor) is low.

8. The F factor can integrate into the host bacterial chromosome, forming an Hfr bacterium. In the process of returning to its independent state, the F factor occasionally excises imprecisely, picking up a piece of the adjacent bacterial chromosome and becoming an F'. When the F' is transferred to a bacterium with a complete chromosome, the recipient cell becomes diploid for the bacterial genes carried on that F'. The cell is said to be a partial diploid, or merozygote.

9. Transformation requires *competence* on the part of the recipient bacterium, meaning that only under certain conditions are bacterial cells capable of being transformed. Transforming DNA must initially be *double-stranded*, yet it is converted to a single-stranded structure during insertion into the host cell. Early transformation studies showed that the most effective size of the transforming DNA is about 10,000 to 20,000 nucleotide pairs. Transformation is an energy-requiring process, and the number of sites on the bacterial cell surface is limited.

10. The phage not only lacks genes for ribosomal construction, but also contains no ribosomes. Upon infection, phage genes are transcribed, and the transcripts are translated using bacterial ribosomes.

11. Details of the life cycle will vary depending on the particular phage under consideration. Here, the life cycle of the T4 phage is described. The life cycle is generally initiated when the virus binds by adsorption to the bacterial host cell. Contraction of the outer sheath causes the central core to breach the cell wall allowing viral DNA in the head to be injected into the bacterium. Synthesis of bacterial DNA, RNA, and protein is inhibited, and degradation of host DNA is initiated. Synthesis of viral molecules, using bacterial machinery, begins: Phage DNA replication occurs and components of the head, tail, and tail fibers are synthesized. From the resulting pools of viral DNA and proteins, phage particles are assembled, using three sequential pathways: DNA is packaged into viral heads; virus tails are assembled; and tail fibers are assembled.

DNA-filled heads combine with the tail components, and the tail fibers are added to complete the assembly of progeny phage.

12. A single plaque originates from the replicative activity of a single bacteriophage.

13. A single plaque is a clearing of bacteria resulting from the lytic action of millions of bacteriophages.

14. Each of the three serial dilutions made is a hundred-fold dilution. The final dilution, therefore, is a $10^{-2} \times 10^{-2} \times 10^{-2} = 10^{-6}$ dilution. Given the introduction of 0.1 mL of the phage dilution to the bacterial suspension, the initial density of

bacteriophage suspension would be calculated as follows:

17 phage/0.1 mL $\times 10^6 = 1.7 \times 10^8$ phage/mL

15. A lytic cycle occurs when a bacteriophage enters a bacterial host, form progeny phages, and lyse the host after a relatively short period of time. There is no extensive latent period.By contrast, in lysogeny, certain temperate phages can enter a bacterial cell and integrate their DNA into the bacterial chromosome instead of following a lytic developmental path. There is an extended latent phase, in which viral DNA is replicated with each bacterial generation, but no progeny phages are produced. At any point, the integrated viral DNA can be induced to excise from the host chromosome, triggering the lytic cycle.

16. A prophage is the latent, noninfective state of the bacteriophage chromosome when it is incorporated into the host bacterial chromosome.

17. In their experiment, Zinder and Lederberg prevented contact between the two auxotrophic strains, by using a Davis U-tube apparatus fitted with a sintered filter. F-mediated conjugation requires cell-to-cell contact, and without it, conjugation cannot occur. Recovery of prototrophic bacteria indicated that a filterable agent (FA) was present, which mediated the gene transfer. The treatment with DNase showed that the filterable agent was not naked DNA.

18. Cotransduction of two or three genes can be used to determine the map order. The cotransduction of two or more bacterial genes is more likely if they appear on the same DNA fragment than if they are located on two separate DNA fragments. The genes are more likely to be found on a single DNA fragment the closer they are to each other on the intact bacterial chromosome.

19. Starting with a single bacteriophage, one lytic cycle produces 200 progeny phages; after three more lytic cycles, $(200)^4$ or 1,600,000,000 phages would be produced.

20. For each plate, assume that a volume of 0.1 mL of phage dilution was used in the plaque assay.

(a) Since all bacteria lysed, the initial concentration of the phage stock is greater than 10^5 phage/mL.

(b) This result indicates that the initial concentration of the phage stock is around $14/0.1 \times 10^6$ or 1.4×10^8 phage/mL.

(c) Because no plaques were detected, the initial concentration of phages is less than 10^9. This is consistent with the calculations performed in part (b).

Chapter 9: DNA Structure and Analysis

Concept Areas	Corresponding Problems
Central Dogma	1, 2, 19, 25
DNA as Genetic Material	1, 2, 3, 4, 5, 6, 7, 8
Transformation	1, 4, 5
Differential Labeling	1, 6, 7
Genetic Variation	2, 28, 29
Model Building	1, 10, 14, 15, 16, 27, 30
Nucleic Acid Structure	1, 2, 6, 7, 10, 11, 12, 13, 14, 15, 16, 17, 18, 24, 25, 26, 28, 29, 31
Analytical Methods	6, 7, 8, 20, 21, 22, 23, 24, 27, 31, 32
Replication	2, 25
RNA as Genetic Material	2, 9

Structures and Processes Checklist—Significant items that deserve special attention are identified with a "*".

(Check topic when mastered–provide examples where appropriate–understand the context of each entry)

- **Overview**
  - genetic material*
  - DNA as informational basis of heredity
  - Watson and Crick*
- **Four Characteristics***
  - replication*
  - storage of information*
  - expression of information*
  - variation by mutation*
  - partitioned by mitosis and meiosis
  - information flow
  - transcription*
  - translation*
  - central dogma of molecular genetics*

- **Observations Favoring Protein**
  - nuclein
  - tetranucleotide hypothesis
- **Evidence Favoring DNA***
  - transformation studies*
  - virulent strains
  - avirulent strains
  - polysaccharide capsule
  - smooth colonies (*S*)
  - rough colonies (*R*)
  - serotypes
  - *Diplococcus* II*R* and III*S*
  - transformation*
  - transforming principle*

- *in vitro*
- Avery, MacLeod, McCarty*
- protease*
- ribonuclease (RNase)*
- deoxyribonuclease (DNase)*
- transformation is hereditable
- bacteriophage T2
- phage
- Hershey–Chase*
- 50 percent protein : 50 percent DNA*
- ^{32}P (DNA), ^{35}S (protein)
- radioactive labeling
- ^{35}S-labeled phage "ghosts"
- ^{32}P-labeled progeny phage*
- protoplasts (spheroplasts)
- transfection*

○ **DNA Is Genetic Material in Eukaryotes**

- indirect evidence*
- subcellular distribution
- correlation with ploidy*
- ultraviolet (UV) light
- action spectrum*
- absorption spectrum*
- mutagenic wavelength correlates with DNA absorption*
- direct evidence*
- recombinant DNA technology
- genomics

○ **RNA as Genetic Material***

- tobacco mosaic virus (TMV)*
- phage Qβ
- RNA replicase
- retrovirus*
- reverse transcription*
- reverse transcriptase
- human immunodeficiency virus (HIV)

○ **Structure of DNA***

- model building*
- nitrogenous base*
- pentose sugar*
- phosphate group*
- purine*
- pyrimidine*
- adenine (A)*
- guanine (G)*
- cytosine (C)*
- thymine (T)*
- uracil (U)*
- ribonucleic acid (RNA)*
- ribose*
- deoxyribonucleic acid (DNA)*
- deoxyribose*
- 2-deoxyribose
- nucleoside
- nucleotide
- nucleoside monophosphate (NMP)
- nucleoside diphosphate (NDP)

- ○ nucleoside triphosphate (NTP)
- ○ adenosine triphosphate (ATP)*
- ○ guanosine triphosphate (GTP)*
- ○ inorganic phosphate (P_i)
- ○ phosphodiester bond*
- ○ oligonucleotides
- ○ polynucleotides
- ○ base composition*
- ○ Chargaff
- ○ proportionality*
- ○ (A + G) = (C + T)*
- ○ X-ray diffraction analysis*
- ○ Watson–Crick model*
- ○ right-handed double helix
- ○ antiparallel
- ○ bases stacked
- ○ bases paired*
- ○ 3.4 nm per turn
- ○ minor groove
- ○ major groove
- ○ 2.0 nm diameter
- ○ complementarity*
- ○ hydrogen bond*
- ○ hydrophobic*
- ○ hydrophilic*
- ○ semiconservative mode of replication*
- ○ **Alternative DNA Forms**
  - ○ A-DNA*
  - ○ B-DNA*
  - ○ single-crystal X-ray analysis
  - ○ Z-DNA*

- ○ left-handed double helix
- ○ zig-zag conformation
- ○ **RNA Structure***
  - ○ ribosomal RNA (rRNA)*
  - ○ messenger RNA (mRNA)*
  - ○ transfer RNA (tRNA)*
  - ○ sedimentation behavior
  - ○ Svedberg coefficient (*S*)
  - ○ ribosomes
  - ○ telomerase RNA
  - ○ small nuclear RNA (snRNA)
  - ○ antisense RNA
  - ○ microRNA (miRNA)
  - ○ short interfering RNA (siRNA)
  - ○ long noncoding RNA (lncRNA)
- ○ **Analytical Techniques***
  - ○ DNA denaturation
  - ○ hyperchromic shift*
  - ○ melting profile
  - ○ melting temperature (T_m)*
  - ○ denaturation/renaturation
  - ○ molecular hybridization*
  - ○ probes*
  - ○ *in situ* molecular hybridization*
  - ○ fluorescence *in situ* hybridization (FISH)*
  - ○ electrophoresis*
  - ○ agarose gel*
  - ○ blotting*

Answers to Now Solve This

9.1 In an *in vitro* transformation experiment, the general differential labeling design of the Hershey–Chase experiment would *theoretically* be appropriate: Some substance, if labeled, could show up in the recipient bacterium or its progeny. However, in practice, there would be complications, chief among them that only one strand is taken up and fragment length is relatively small compared to the genomic DNA of the recipient bacterium. As a result, the majority of the ^{32}P label would be recovered outside the cell, and any DNA that did enter the cell would be difficult to detect. Overall, this could potentially lead to the conclusion that the ^{32}P-labeled material (DNA) was unable to enter recipient cells.

9.2 Guanine = 17.5 percent, adenine and thymine each = 32.5 percent.

9.3 Because uracil is present rather than thymine, the genetic material is RNA. Assuming the value of 1.13 is statistically different from 1.00, purines outnumber pyrimidines; therefore, the nucleic acid is single-stranded. Overall, one can conclude that rubella is a single-stranded RNA virus.

Chapter 9 DNA Structure and Analysis

Solutions to Problems and Discussion Questions

1. (a) Key evidence that DNA is the genetic material originally came from experiments using bacteria and bacteriophages. Transformation studies showed that DNA is the genetic material in bacteria and differential labeling (proteins and nucleic acids) of bacteriophage T2 showed that DNA is the genetic material in some viruses. Both direct and indirect studies have shown that DNA is the genetic material in eukaryotes. Other than in mitochondria and chloroplasts, DNA is localized in the nucleus, where its quantity varies with ploidy (n, $2n$), as one would predict for the genetic material. In addition, the action spectrum of UV light overlaps the absorption spectrum of DNA (see text Figure 9.5). Direct evidence comes from recombinant DNA studies in which transgenic organisms can be generated with transferred DNA as well as genomics analysis.

(b) A right-handed double helix with antiparallel polynucleotide chains was first proposed by Watson and Crick based on the X-ray diffraction studies of Franklin and Wilkins. The constant diameter of the DNA double helix and its greatest stability in a right-handed form add additional support.

(c) Given base composition studies showing proportional amounts of A and T, and G and C, and X-ray diffraction studies, Watson and Crick showed that hydrogen bonding configurations between the bases provided attraction and stability for a DNA double helix.

2. Your essay should include a description of structural aspects, including sugar and base content comparisons. In addition, you should mention complementation aspects, strandedness, flexibility, and conformation.

3. Prior to 1940, most of the interest in genetics centered on the transmission of similarity and variation from parents to offspring (transmission genetics). While some experiments examined the possible nature of the hereditary material, abundant knowledge of the structural and enzymatic properties of proteins generated a bias that worked to favor proteins as the hereditary substance.

In addition, proteins were composed of as many as 20 different subunits (amino acids), thereby providing ample structural and functional variation for the multiple tasks that must be accomplished by the genetic material. The tetranucleotide hypothesis, which postulated that DNA consisted of a set of four repeated nucleotide components, provided insufficient variability to account for the diverse roles of the genetic material.

4. Griffith was the first to observe (and name) the phenomenon of transformation, using an *in vivo* system (laboratory mice). He observed that a bacterial mixture containing heat-killed cells of a virulent strain of *Diplococcus pneumoniae* and live cells of an avirulent strain killed the injected mice and led to recovery of live cells of the virulent strain. He concluded that the heat-killed virulent bacteria transformed the avirulent strain into a virulent strain. Although he did not identify the "transforming principle," he did propose that it might be some component of the polysaccharide capsule (the one visible difference between the two strains). By contrast, Avery and coworkers, using an *in vitro* system, systematically searched for the transforming principle originating from the heat-killed pathogenic strain and determined it to be DNA.

5. Avery and colleagues isolated the "transforming principle" as a bacterial extract that consisted of a mixture of macromolecules. To identify which macromolecule was, in fact, the transforming principle, specific degradative enzymes (proteases, RNase, and DNase) were used to selectively eliminate components of the extract. The rationale was that if transformation were concomitantly eliminated, then the eliminated component would be the transforming principle. Only DNase, which eliminated DNA, prevented transformation; therefore, DNA must be the transforming principle.

6. Nucleic acids contain large amounts of phosphorus and no sulfur, whereas proteins contain sulfur and no phosphorus. Therefore, the radioisotopes ^{32}P and ^{35}S will selectively label nucleic acids and proteins, respectively.

The Hershey–Chase experiment was based on the premise that the substance injected by the bacteriophage into the bacterium is the substance responsible for producing the progeny phages and, therefore, must be the hereditary material. The experiment demonstrated that most of the ^{32}P-labeled material (phage DNA) was injected, whereas the ^{35}S-labeled phage ghosts (phage protein coats) remained outside the bacterium. Furthermore, progeny phage contained the ^{32}P label and not the ^{35}S label. Therefore, the nucleic acid must be the genetic material.

7. Phosphorus is found in approximately equal amounts in DNA and RNA. Therefore, labeling with ^{32}P would "tag" both RNA and DNA. However, the T2 phage, in its mature state, contains very little, if any, RNA; therefore, DNA would be interpreted as being the genetic material in the T2 phage.

8. The early evidence would be considered indirect. The location of DNA only in subcellular structures where genetic functions occur (the nucleus, chloroplasts and mitochondria) favored DNA over proteins as the genetic information. Further indirect evidence came from the observation that DNA content and ploidy in various cell types (sperm and somatic cells) were related. Moreover, the correlation of the *action* and *absorption* spectra of ultraviolet light supported the interpretation that DNA was the genetic material. Direct evidence for DNA being the genetic material comes from a variety of observations, including gene transfer, which has been facilitated by recombinant DNA techniques.

9. Some viruses contain a genetic material composed of RNA. The tobacco mosaic virus (TMV) is composed of an RNA core and a protein coat. Spreading purified TMV RNA on tobacco leaves resulted in the formation of characteristic TMV lesions. Retroviruses contain RNA as the genetic material and use an enzyme known as *reverse transcriptase* to produce DNA, which can be integrated into the host chromosome. See F1.1 in Chapter 1 of this study guide.

10. The structure of deoxyadenylic acid is given in the following diagram and in the text. Linkages among the three components require the removal of water (H_2O).

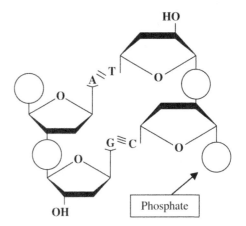

11. The numbering of the carbons on the sugar is especially important (see the following diagram). Examine the text (Figure 9.6) for the numbers on the carbons and nitrogens of the bases.

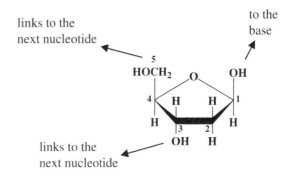

12. Examine the structures of the bases in the text. The other bases would be named as follows:

Guanine:	2-amino-6-oxypurine
Cytosine:	2-oxy-4-aminopyrimidine
Thymine:	2, 4-dioxy-5-methylpyrimidine
Uracil:	2, 4-dioxypyrimidine

13. Examine the text [Figure 9.11(c)] for the format for this drawing. Note that the complementary strand must be drawn in the antiparallel orientation.

14. The following are characteristics of the Watson–Crick double-helix model for DNA:

There are two antiparallel polynucleotide chains, which coil around each other to form a double helix. Each chain is formed by phosphodiester linkages between the five-carbon sugars and the phosphates. Bases are stacked, 0.34 nm apart with 10 bases per turn. Hydrogen bonds hold the two polynucleotide chains together. There are two hydrogen bonds between the A-T pair and three between the G-C pair. The double helix is approximately 2 nm in diameter, with a topography of major and minor grooves. The hydrophobic bases are located in the center of the molecule, whereas the hydrophilic phosphodiester backbone is on the outside.

15. Watson and Crick knew the chemical structure of each nitrogenous base and of each nucleoside. They also had available the X-ray diffraction information of Astbury, Franklin, and Wilkins and the base ratio information of Chargaff. Their approach was to construct a "simple" model that would account for the known chemical and physical properties and have a natural beauty in its simplicity.

16. The data given show that A = C and T = G. However, in the most common forms of these bases, opposite charge relationships do not exist between A and C nor between T and G, so pairing would not occur. This would make it unlikely that a tight helical structure would form. This observation would likely lead to the interpretation of DNA as a single-stranded or other nonhydrogen-bonded structure. Such structures would not produce the regular X-ray diffraction pattern observed by Wilkins and Franklin, which indicated a double-helical structure.

17. A covalent bond is a relatively strong bond that involves the sharing of electrons between two or more atoms. Hydrogen bonds, which are much weaker than covalent bonds, are formed as a result of electrostatic attraction between a covalently bonded hydrogen atom and an atom with an unshared electron pair. The hydrogen atom assumes a partial positive charge, while the unshared electron pair—characteristic of covalently bonded oxygen and nitrogen atoms—assumes a partial negative charge. These opposite charges are responsible for the weak chemical attraction.

Complementarity is based on hydrogen bonding and is responsible for the chemical attraction between adenine and thymine (uracil in RNA) and guanine and cytosine. This results in DNA and, to a limited extent, RNA, assuming a double-stranded conformation.

18. Three main differences between RNA and DNA are the following:

(1) Uracil in RNA replaces thymine in DNA.
(2) Ribose in RNA replaces deoxyribose in DNA.
(3) RNA often occurs as both single- and partially double-stranded forms, whereas DNA most often occurs in a double-stranded form.

19. Although there are many types of RNA, the three main types described in this section are presented next:

Ribosomal RNA: rRNA combines with proteins to form ribosomes, which function to align mRNA and charged tRNA molecules during translation.

Transfer RNA: tRNAs are involved in protein synthesis in that they represent a "link" between the coding sequences in DNA (as reflected in mRNA) and the ordering of amino acids in proteins. Transfer RNAs are specific in that each species is attached to only one type of amino acid.

Messenger RNA: The coding sequences in DNA are relayed to the site of protein synthesis by relatively short-lived molecules called messenger RNAs. In eukaryotes, mRNA carries genetic information from the nucleus to the cytoplasm. It is the sequence of bases in mRNA that specifies the order of amino acids in proteins.

20. The nitrogenous bases of nucleic acids absorb UV light maximally at wavelengths of 254 to 260 nm. Using this phenomenon, one can often determine the presence and concentration of nucleic acids in mixtures of biologically important molecules. UV absorption is greater in single-stranded DNA molecules as compared with double-stranded structures (hyperchromic shift); therefore, by applying denaturing conditions, one can easily determine whether a nucleic acid is in the single- or double-stranded form. In addition, A-T rich DNA denatures more readily than G-C rich DNA. Therefore, one can estimate base content by denaturation kinetics.

21. High temperatures disrupt the hydrogen bonds that hold together the complementary strands of DNA, causing double-stranded DNA to become single stranded.

22. A *hyperchromic effect* is the increased absorption of UV light as double-stranded DNA (or RNA) is converted to a single-stranded form. As illustrated in the text, the change in absorption is quite significant, with structures of higher G-C content *melting* at higher temperatures than A-T rich nucleic acids. If one monitors the UV absorption with a spectrophotometer during the melting process, the hyperchromic shift can be observed. The T_m is the point (temperature) on the profile at which half (50 percent) of the sample is denatured.

23. G-C base pairs are formed with three hydrogen bonds whereas A-T base pairs by two such bonds.

Therefore, it takes more energy (higher temperature) to separate G-C pairs.

24. The association (or reassociation) of separate complementary strands of a nucleic acid, either DNA or RNA, is based on the formation of hydrogen bonds between A-T (or U) and G-C.

25. In one sentence of their first *Nature* paper, Watson and Crick state,

> It has not escaped our notice that the specific pairing we have postulated immediately suggests a possible copying mechanism for the genetic material.

The model itself indicates that unwinding of the helix and separation of the double-stranded structure into two single strands immediately expose the specific hydrogen bonds through which new bases are brought into place.

26. (1) As shown, the extra phosphate is not normally expected.

(2) In the adenine ring, a nitrogen is at position 8 rather than position 9, and a carbon is at position 9 rather than position 8.

(3) The bond from the C-1' of the sugar should form with the N at position 9 (N-9) of the adenine.

(4) There should be a double bond between C-4 and C-5 of adenine.

(5) The dinucleotide is a "deoxy" form; therefore, each C-2' should not have a hydroxyl group. Notice the hydroxyl group at C-2' on the sugar of the adenylic acid.

(6) At the C-5 position on the thymine residue, there should be a methyl group.

(7) There are too many bonds between the N-3 and C-2 of thymine.

(8) There are too few bonds between the C-5 and C-6 of thymine (there should be a double bond there).

(9) The extra hydroxyl group on C-5' of the sugar of the thymidylic acid should not be there (the C-5' hydroxyl group is involved in the bond with the phosphate group).

27. **(a)** The similarity of the X-ray diffraction pattern to that of DNA would suggest a helical structure for this new nucleic acid. The irregularities may indicate different diameters along the helix, additional strands in the helix, kinking, or bending.

(b) The hyperchromic shift indicates base pairing, caused by considerable hydrogen bonding.

(c) The base composition data indicate that all the bases presented are purines. This suggests irregular base pairing in which purines bind purines, which could account for the atypical dimensions. In addition, the unequal proportions of adenine and hypoxanthine suggest there may be some single-stranded components.

(d) One-quarter of the sugar residues were identified as ribose, suggesting that the molecule may show more flexibility, kinking, and/or folding than does DNA.

Although several situations are possible for this model, the phosphates are still likely to be on the outside of the helix and well separated from each other because of their strong like charges. The nitrogenous bases probably exists on the inside of the molecule, stabilized by hydrogen bonding. The molecule is also likely to display considerable flexibility, kinking, and/or bending.

28. Assuming the lesion is not repaired, the result would be a base substitution of G-C to A-T after two rounds of replication, because the original cytosine pairing with guanine would be replaced with uracil pairing with adenine.

29. Under this condition, the hydrolyzed 5-methyl cytosine becomes thymine.

30. **(a, b)** Given the chemical similarities to terrestrial DNA, it is probable that the unique creature's DNA follows a similar structural plan. The X-ray diffraction pattern suggests a wider helix than terrestrial DNA. Because there are equal amounts of A, T, and H, one could suggest that they are hydrogen bonded to one another; the same may be said for C, G, and X. Given the molar equivalence of erythrose and phosphate, an alternating sugar-phosphate-sugar backbone, would seem likely. A model of a triple helix would be consistent with these data.

(c) Hypoxanthine and xanthine each interact with a purine-pyrimidine pair. To achieve the constant diameter indicated, both would need to be of the same class, either purine or pyrimidine (as also suggested by the similarity of their names). In fact, hypoxanthine and xanthine are both purines.

31. (i) Heat application would yield a hyperchromic shift if the DNA is double-stranded. One could also get a rough estimation of the G-C content from the kinetics of denaturation.

(ii) Determination of base content could be used for comparative purposes and could also provide evidence as to the strandedness of the DNA.

(iii) X-ray crystallography would indicate whether the DNA has a helical structure and single-crystal X-ray analysis would reveal even greater structural detail.

(iv) Agarose gel electrophoresis would allow determination of the size of each viral DNA, which could then be compared.

(v) Labeled probes could be made from the DNA of each virus and used in reciprocal *in situ* molecular hybridization studies to determine whether there are similarities at the sequence level.

(vi) Sequencing the DNA from both viruses would indicate specific sequence homology. In addition, through various electronic searches readily available on the Internet (*www.ncbi.nlm.nih.gov*, for example), one could determine whether similar sequences exist in other viruses or in other organisms.

32. Even though RNA molecules, like DNA molecules, have the same charge-to-mass ratios, they are single-stranded and can exist in a variety of shapes. Complementary intrastrand base pairing can make more compact structures compared to the more relaxed, open conformation of molecules that do not base pair. As with DNA, during electrophoresis, smaller and more compact molecules migrate faster than do relaxed, open structures. Therefore, RNA molecules must be denatured to eliminate secondary structural variables in order to perform electrophoretic size comparisons.

Chapter 10: DNA Replication

Concept Areas	Corresponding Problems
In Vitro Experiments	1, 3, 4, 5, 7, 8, 9, 22
Mode of Replication	3, 4, 5, 6, 22
General Replication	2, 10, 14, 15, 16, 17
Replication in Bacteria	1, 4, 7, 8, 9, 11, 12, 13, 18, 20, 21
Replication in Eukaryotes	1, 5, 18, 23, 24
Base Composition	8, 19
Enzymology	1, 7, 8, 9, 10, 11, 12, 13, 15, 16, 17, 20, 21
Replication mutants	1, 9, 11, 20, 21
Telomerase	1, 23, 24

Structures and Processes Checklist—Significant items that deserve special attention are identified with a "*".

(Check topic when mastered–provide examples where appropriate–understand the context of each entry)

- o **Overview**
  - o mode of replication
  - o details of DNA synthesis
- o **Semiconservative Replication***
  - o each DNA strand as template
  - o complementarity*
  - o semiconservative replication*
  - o conservative replication*
  - o dispersive replication*
  - o Meselson–Stahl Experiment*
  - o replication in bacteria
  - o $^{15}NH_4Cl$ (ammonium chloride)*
  - o heavy isotope
  - o sedimentation equilibrium centrifugation*
  - o ^{15}N-DNA*
  - o "new" DNA incorporated lighter isotope

- o intermediate density*
- o replication in eukaryotes*
- o Taylor, Woods, Hughes*
- o radioactive thymidine*
- o autoradiography*
- o "grains"
- o origin of replication
- o unidirectional* or bidirectional*?
- o replication fork
- o replicon
- o *E. coli*
- o *oriC*
- o *ter**
- o **Five Bacterial Polymerases***
  - o DNA polymerase I*
  - o *in vitro* DNA synthesis
  - o addition at the 3'-OH end*

- ○ chain elongation
- ○ 5' to 3' direction*
- ○ fidelity
- ○ *polA1* mutant strain*
- ○ susceptibility to DNA damage
- ○ DNA polymerases II and III
- ○ primer*
- ○ 3′ to 5′ exonuclease activity
- ○ proofreading capacity
- ○ 5′ to 3′ exonuclease activity of DNA polymerase I
- ○ removal of primer
- ○ DNA polymerases IV and V
- ○ repair enzymes
- ○ holoenzyme
- ○ core enzyme
- ○ sliding clamp loader
- ○ sliding DNA clamp
- ○ processivity*
- ○ **Complex Issues***
  - ○ unwinding the helix
  - ○ *oriC*
  - ○ 9mers
  - ○ 13mers
  - ○ DnaA (initiator protein)
  - ○ DNA helicase (DnaB polypeptide)*
  - ○ single-stranded binding proteins (SSBs)
  - ○ supercoiling
  - ○ DNA gyrase
  - ○ DNA topoisomerases
  - ○ replisome*
  - ○ initiation of DNA synthesis*
  - ○ RNA primer*
  - ○ primase*
- ○ antiparallel*
- ○ continuous DNA synthesis
- ○ leading strand*
- ○ discontinuous synthesis*
- ○ lagging strand*
- ○ semidiscontinuous synthesis*
- ○ Okazaki fragments*
- ○ DNA ligase
- ○ *lig* mutant strain
- ○ concurrent synthesis*
- ○ looping of lagging strand template*
- ○ proofreading*
- ○ **Coherent Model***
  - ○ summary of the process of bacterial DNA replication
- ○ **Genes Control Replication ***
  - ○ conditional mutations*
  - ○ temperature-sensitive mutation
  - ○ permissive
  - ○ restrictive
- ○ **Eukaryotic DNA Replication***
  - ○ shares many features with replication in bacteria
  - ○ greater amounts of DNA
  - ○ nucleosomes
  - ○ linear chromosomes
  - ○ multiple origins
  - ○ slower synthesis rate
  - ○ autonomously replicating sequences (ARSs)*
  - ○ consensus sequence*
  - ○ multiple eukaryotic polymerases
  - ○ Pol α enzyme
  - ○ processivity*
  - ○ polymerase switching*

- Pol ε–leading strand
- Pol δ–lagging strand
- Pol γ–mitochondrial DNA
- replication through chromatin
- chromatin assembly factors (CAFs)

○ **Eukaryotic Chromosome Ends***

- double-stranded breaks (DSBs)
- telomeres*
- G-rich strand
- C-rich strand
- t-loops
- shelterin complex
- replication at telomers*

- end-replication problem
- telomerase*
- ribonucleoprotein
- telomerase RNA component (TERC)
- reverse transcription*
- telomerase reverse transcriptase (TERT)
- telomeres, disease, and aging
- limited telomerase expression
- somatic cell telomere erosion
- senescence
- alternative lengthening of telomeres (ALT)

F10.1 Shorthand structures for 3' and 5' nucleotides.

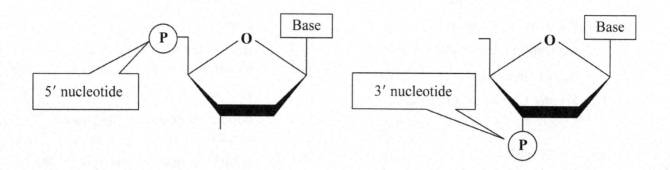

F10.2 Illustration of the influence of a conditional mutation on protein structure and function.

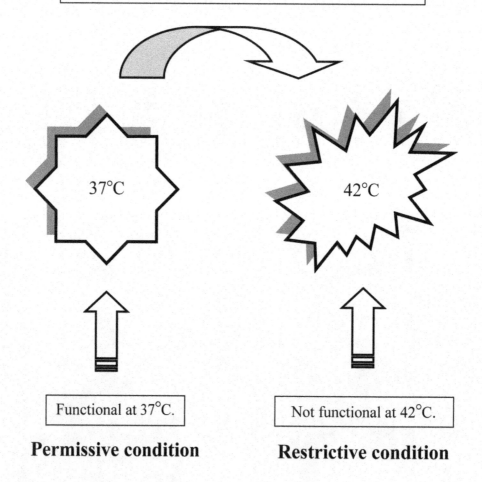

Changes in the environment of the protein may cause conformational changes in the protein to alter function of that protein.

37°C

42°C

Functional at 37°C.

Not functional at 42°C.

Permissive condition

Restrictive condition

F10.3 This figure relating to question 5 in the problems section depicts labeling patterns under *conservative* and *dispersive* replication patterns.

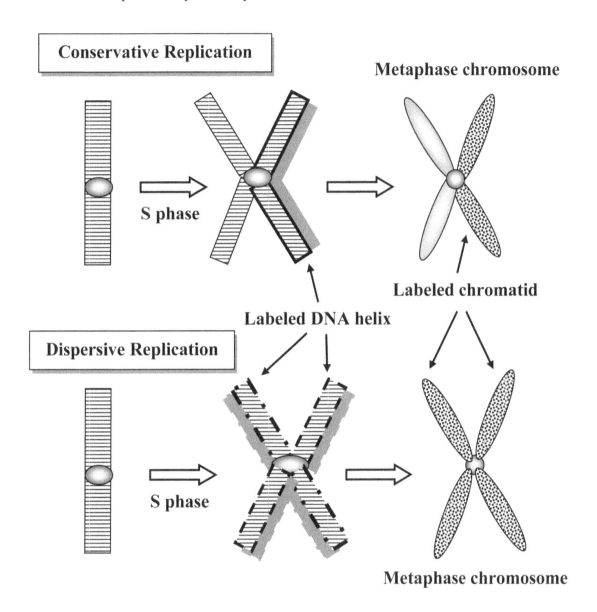

Answers to Now Solve This

10.1 Under a conservative scheme, the first round of replication in ^{14}N medium produces one dense double helix and one light double helix, in contrast to the intermediate density of the DNA in the semiconservative mode. Therefore, after one round of replication in the ^{14}N medium, the conservative scheme can be ruled out. After one round of replication in ^{14}N under a dispersive model, the DNA would be of intermediate density, just as it is in the semiconservative model. However, after the second round of dispersive replication in ^{14}N medium, DNA molecules would be of an intermediate density, with a ratio of ^{15}N:^{14}N less than that after one round of replication. This contrasts with the observation that DNA molecules are of either intermediate or light density after two generations. Therefore, the dispersive mode is ruled out after two rounds of replication.

10.2 If the DNA double helix contained parallel (rather than antiparallel) strands and if the polymerase were able to accommodate such parallel strands, there would be continuous synthesis and no Okazaki fragments. Several other possibilities exist: The DNA existed only as a single strand; synthesis was initiated from two origins located at opposite ends of a linear molecule, producing a continuous complementary strand for each template; this could also occur from a single origin on a circular molecule.

Chapter 10 DNA Replication

Solutions to Problems and Discussion Questions

1. (a) Two classic experiments, one using *E. coli* and the other using *Vicia faba*, using density and radioisotope labeling, respectively, demonstrated that replication is semiconservative in bacteria and eukaryotes. In both cases, daughter DNA molecules are each composed of one parental strand and one newly synthesized DNA strand.

(b) A mutant in DNA polymerase I (*polA1*) was nevertheless capable of synthesizing biologically active DNA, leading to the conclusion that at least one other enzyme is responsible for replicating DNA *in vivo*.

(c) *In vitro* studies by Kornberg and coworkers indicated that DNA strand elongation occurs by addition of nucleotides at the 3' end. During chain elongation, two of the outer phosphates of the precursor dNTP are cleaved, and the remaining phosphate attaches to the 3'-OH group of the deoxyribose. *In vivo* or *in vitro*, DNA polymerases, including polymerase III, are capable only of 5' to 3' synthesis.

(d) Two lines of evidence indicated that DNA synthesis is discontinuous. First, in newly formed DNA, relatively short nucleotide fragments are hydrogen bonded to the template strands. Second, these short nucleotide fragments accumulate in ligase-deficient mutants of *E. coli*.

(e) Because eukaryotic chromosomes are linear rather than circular, free ends exist. It was predicted that such free ends would create the problem of chromosome shortening because of the 5' to 3' nature of DNA synthesis and the inability of DNA polymerases to initiate synthesis without a free 3'-OH. The finding of the telomerase enzyme and a number of terminal repeats at the ends of chromosomes provided support for the prediction of chromosome shortening and also provided its solution.

2. Your essay should describe replication as the process of making daughter nucleic acids from existing ones. Synthesis refers to the precise series of steps, components, and reactions that allow such replication to occur.

3. The differences among the three models of DNA replication relate to the manner in which the new strands of DNA are oriented as daughter DNA molecules are produced.

Conservative: The original double helix remains as a complete unit and the new DNA double helix is produced as a single unit. The old DNA is completely conserved.

Semiconservative: Each daughter molecule is composed of one old DNA strand and one new DNA strand. Strand separation in the template molecule by disruption of hydrogen bonds is required.

Dispersive: The original DNA strand is broken into pieces and the new DNA in the daughter strand is interspersed among the old pieces. Breakage of the individual covalent phosphodiester bonds is required for this mode of replication.

4. By uniformly labeling the nitrogenous bases of the DNA of *E. coli* with the heavy isotope ^{15}N, it was possible to "follow" the "old" (parental) DNA. This was accomplished by growing the cells for many generations in medium containing ^{15}N. Cells were transferred to ^{14}N medium so that "new" (daughter) DNA could be detected. A comparison of the density of DNA samples removed at various times in the experiment (initial ^{15}N culture and subsequent cultures grown in the ^{14}N medium) showed that after one round of replication in the ^{14}N medium, the DNA was half as dense (intermediate) as the DNA from bacteria grown only in the ^{15}N medium. In a sample taken after two rounds of replication in the ^{14}N medium, half of the DNA was of the intermediate density, and the other half was as dense as DNA containing only ^{14}N DNA.

5. Refer to the text for an illustration of the labeling of *Vicia* chromosomes under a Taylor, Woods, and Hughes experimental design. Notice that only those cells that pass through the S phase in the presence of the ^{3}H-thymidine are labeled and that, in each double helix (per chromatid), only one of the two strands is labeled (that is, each chromatid is "half-labeled").

(a) Under a conservative scheme, after the first round of synthesis, one sister chromatid would consist entirely of newly synthesized DNA, with label on both strands of the double helix, whereas the other sister chromatid will remain the original unlabeled parent double helix. (See F10.3 in this handbook.)

(b) Under a dispersive scheme, all of the newly labeled DNA will be interspersed with unlabeled DNA. In preparations of metaphase chromosomes, the structures are highly coiled and condensed, so it would be impossible to detect the areas where labeling is not found. Rather, both sister chromatids would appear as evenly labeled structures (F10.3 in this handbook). This would be similar to the results seen for semiconservative replication. However, after a second round of replication (this time in unlabeled medium) using a dispersive scheme, again, both sister chromatids will be labeled. This outcome contrasts with the result in a semiconservative scheme, in which only one sister chromatid would be labeled and the other unlabeled.

6. The model proposed a triple helical DNA structure. Because the semiconservative scheme predicts that *half* of the DNA in each daughter double helix is labeled, it would be difficult to envision a scheme in which three strands are replicated in such a semiconservative manner. It is possible that either the conservative or dispersive scheme would fit more appropriately. To examine the nature of replication, one could devise an experiment similar to that of Meselson and Stahl or of Taylor, Woods, and Hughes.

7. The *in vitro* replication requires a DNA template, a primer to provide a free 3′-OH, a divalent cation (Mg^{2+}), and all four of the deoxyribonucleoside triphosphates: dATP, dCTP, dTTP, and dGTP.

8. The indirect approach described in the text was the analysis of *base composition*. Comparison of the bases comprising the template with those of the product showed that, within experimental error, expectations were met and that the DNA replicated faithfully.

9. DeLucia and Cairns discovered a strain of *E. coli* (*polA1*) that still replicates its DNA but is deficient in DNA polymerase I activity. Furthermore, DNA Pol I is capable of degrading as well as synthesizing DNA, which suggested that it functions more as a repair than a replicative enzyme.

10. An exposed 3′-OH group is a direct participant in the attachment of the next nucleotide. The oxygen atom of the free 3′-hydroxyl forms a covalent bond with the 5′-phosphate of the incoming nucleotide, which results in the release of inorganic pyrophosphate.

11. The *polA1* mutation was instrumental in demonstrating that DNA polymerase I activity was not necessary for the *in vivo* replication of the *E. coli* chromosome. Such an observation opened the door for the discovery of other enzymes involved in DNA replication.

12. All three enzymes share several properties. First, none can *initiate* DNA synthesis on a template but all can *elongate* an existing DNA strand, assuming there is a template strand as shown in the following figure. Polymerization of nucleotides occurs in the 5′ to 3′ direction; each 5′ phosphate is added to the 3′ end of the growing polynucleotide.

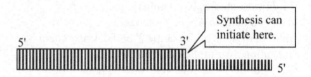

In addition, each enzyme has 3′ to 5′ exonuclease activity, which provides proofreading capabilities. DNA Pol I is unique in its possession of 5′ to 3′ exonuclease activity, which is suitable for its role in removal of RNA primers. Pol I is highly abundant and stable, whereas Pol III is not. Pol I is a single polypeptide, whereas Pol III consists of multiple subunits and is required for chromosomal replication. DNA pol II is believed to be involved in repair synthesis. Refer to the text.

13. Refer to the text for a listing of the components of DNA polymerase III. The active form of the enzyme is called the holoenzyme. The region responsible for actual polymerization is called the "core" portion.

14. (a) After initiation at a given point, *unidirectional* synthesis replicates strands in one direction only, whereas *bidirectional* synthesis replicates strands in both directions. Please refer to the accompanying illustration.

(b) Synthesis using the leading strand template proceeds in the direction of the replication fork and produces a long, unbroken complementary strand and is said to be *continuous*. Synthesis using the lagging strand template proceeds in the direction opposite that of the replication fork and produces multiple, short fragments (Okazaki fragments) that must be ligated together to form a long complementary strand. This type of synthesis is said to be *discontinuous*.

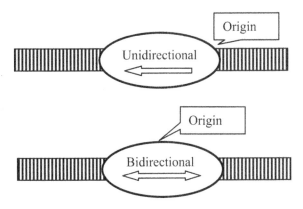

15. *DnaA* binds to AT-rich regions of *oriC* to initiate strand unwinding. *Helicase* uses the energy of ATP hydrolysis to unwind DNA strands, which are then stabilized by *single-stranded DNA-binding proteins*. *DNA gyrase*, a DNA topoisomerase, relieves supercoiling generated by helix unwinding. This process results in separation of the strands of the double helix.

16. (a) Okazaki fragments are relatively short DNA fragments (1000 to 2000 bases in bacteria) that are synthesized in a discontinuous fashion on the lagging strand during DNA replication. Such fragments appear to be necessary because template DNA is not available for 5′ to 3′ synthesis until some degree of continuous DNA synthesis occurs on the leading strand in the direction of the replication fork. The isolation of such fragments provides support for the scheme of replication shown in the text.

(b) DNA ligase is required to form phosphodiester linkages in nicks that are generated when DNA polymerase I removes an RNA primer and meets newly synthesized DNA ahead of it. This action seals the two strands together to form a continuous single strand.

(c) Primer RNA is formed by primase to serve as an initiation point for the production of DNA strands on a DNA template. None of the DNA polymerases are capable of initiating synthesis without a free 3′-hydroxyl group. The primer RNA provides that group and thus can be used by DNA polymerase III.

17. The DNA helix is opened by the initiator protein and helicase and stabilized by single-strand binding proteins. DNA gyrase relieves supercoils generated by DNA unwinding. Next, an RNA primer is synthesized to provide a starting point for DNA polymerase. Replication—the elongation from RNA primers in continuous and discontinuous 5′ to 3′ modes—proceeds in both directions. Primers are removed from both strands by the exonucleolytic activity of DNA polymerase I; Okazaki fragments are joined together with DNA ligase.

18. The increased complexity of the eukaryotic genome led to the expectation that DNA synthesis would also be more complex. First, there is a much greater amount of DNA to be replicated in eukaryotes, and the rate of synthesis by eukaryotic polymerases is much slower than for their bacterial counterparts. These complications are offset by the use of multiple replication origins and the presence of increased levels of DNA polymerase per cell, in contrast to the single replication origin and relatively low levels of polymerase in bacteria. Second, the packaging of eukaryotic DNA into chromosomes adds the complication of replicating around nucleosomes and other proteins, which must be removed before replication and then rapidly reassembled afterward. Histone synthesis is coupled to DNA synthesis to provide sufficient precursors to new nucleosomes. In addition, chromatin assembly factors are present at replication forks. Finally, most eukaryotic chromosomes are linear and will leave single-stranded gaps at the ends of molecules after the removal of RNA primers. Enzymes such as telomerase are therefore needed to replicate the telomeres, or ends of chromosomes.

Eukaryotic DNA is generally replicated in a manner that is very similar to that of *E. coli*. Synthesis is bidirectional, continuous on one strand and discontinuous on the other, and the requirements of synthesis (four deoxyribonucleoside triphosphates, divalent cation, template, and primer) are the same. Okazaki fragments of eukaryotes are about one-tenth the size of those in bacteria.

19. Even though the base composition of two species may be similar, *sequences* can vary considerably.

20. (a) No repair from DNA polymerase I and/or DNA polymerase III

(b) No DNA polymerase I activity and/or no DNA ligase activity

(c) No primase activity; other possibilities include no DnaA protein or faulty helicase

(d) Only DNA polymerase I activity (recall that DNA Pol III has high processivity due to the sliding clamp subunit)

(e) No DNA gyrase activity

21. (a) The α subunit, part of the DNA polymerase III core enzyme, is responsible for DNA synthesis along the template strand. Without this subunit, the cell would not be able to replicate its chromosome. Strains that are mutant for this enzyme contain conditional mutations and can be grown at the permissive condition. Alternatively, mutant cells may rely on DNA polymerase I and replicate their DNA more slowly.

(b) The ε subunit, also part of the DNA polymerase III core enzyme, is responsible for the 3′ to 5′ exonuclease activity that is involved in proofreading. Proofreading would be hampered in such mutant strains and a higher-than-expected mutation rate would occur.

22. If replication is conservative, the first autoradiograms (see "Metaphase" in the text figure) would have labels distributed on only one side (in one chromatid) of the metaphase chromosome, as follows:

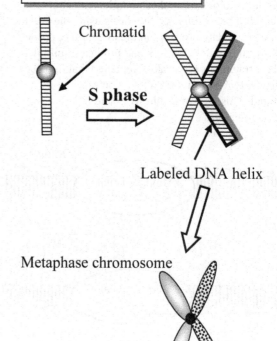

Conservative replication

Chromatid

S phase

Labeled DNA helix

Metaphase chromosome

Labeled chromatid

23. The end-replication problem refers to the difficulties posed in replicating the ends of linear eukaryotic chromosomes. Once primers are removed from the 5′ ends, a gap remains, which cannot be filled. This shortens the chromosome with each round of replication, potentially leading to deletion of gene-coding regions. The action of telomerase lengthens the telomere, which is then made double-stranded (except for the end) through conventional DNA synthesis.

24. Telomerase activity is present in germ-line tissue to maintain telomere length from one generation to the next. It is also necessary in stem cells and other proliferating tissues. In other words, telomeres cannot shorten indefinitely without eventually eroding genetic information.

Chapter 11: Chromosome Structure and DNA Sequence Organization

Concept Areas	Corresponding Problems
Viral and Bacterial Chromosomes	1, 2, 3, 7, 16, 17, 19
Mitochondrial and Chloroplast DNA	3
Specialized Chromosomes	1, 4, 5, 6
Organization of DNA in Chromatin	1, 7, 8, 9, 10, 11, 12, 13, 15
Organization of the Eukaryotic Genome	2, 7, 12, 13, 14, 18

Structures and Processes Checklist—Significant items that deserve special attention are identified with a "*".

(Check topic when mastered–provide examples where appropriate–understand the context of each entry)

- **Overview**
  - organization affects storage, expression, and regulation
  - chromosome structure
  - visual and molecular techniques
  - specialized eukaryotic structures
  - chromatin structure
- **Viral and Bacterial Chromosomes***
  - DNA or RNA
  - linear or circular
  - single- or double-stranded
  - φXI74 bacteriophage
  - polyoma virus
  - bacteriophage lambda (λ)*
  - packaging
  - nucleoid
  - DNA-binding proteins
  - HU protein
  - H-NS (histone-like nucleoid structuring) protein
- **Mitochondrial and Chloroplast DNA***
  - mitochondria*
  - chloroplasts*
  - maternal inheritance*
  - mitochondrial DNA (mtDNA)*
  - varied sizes
  - introns mostly absent*
  - little repetitive DNA
  - little to no intergenic spacer
  - vertebrate mtDNA*
  - strand density differences
  - chloroplast DNA (cpDNA)*
  - size uniformity
  - larger than mtDNA
  - long noncoding introns*

- mtDNA and cpDNA similar to bacterial DNA

- **Specialized Chromosomes***

  - polytene chromosomes*

  - chromomeres

  - replication without strand separation

  - puff*

  - differential gene activity

  - lampbrush chromosome*

  - first prophase of meiosis*

  - Central Axis

  - lateral loops

  - transcriptionally active

- **DNA in Chromatin***

  - chromatin

  - histones*

  - nonhistones

  - five histone types

  - micrococcal nuclease

  - electron microscopy*

  - repeating unit

  - nucleosomes*

  - histone tetramers*

  - $(H2A)_2 \cdot (H2B)_2$ and $(H3)_2 \cdot (H4)_2$

  - nucleosome core particle

  - linker DNA

  - H1

  - solenoid

  - looped domains*

  - coiled chromatin fibers

- packing ratio

- DNA accessibility

- chromatin remodeling*

- histone tails

- acetylation*

- histone acetyltransferase (HAT)

- gene activation

- methylation*

- methyltransferase

- phosphorylation*

- kinase

- 5-methyl cytosine

- CpG island

- epigenetics

- euchromatin*

- heterochromatin*

- position effect

- chromosome banding*

- G-banding

- C-banding

- **Complex Sequence Organization***

  - repetitive DNA*

  - multiple-copy genes

  - satellite DNA*

  - highly repetitive DNA*

  - *in situ* hybridization*

  - centromere*

  - CEN region

  - kinetochore*

  - alphoid family

- CENP-A

- middle (or moderately) repetitive DNA

- variable number tandem repeats (VNTRs)*

- minisatellites*

- DNA fingerprinting*

- microsatellites*

- short tandem repeats (STRs)*

- transposable elements*

- short interspersed elements (SINEs)*

- *Alu* family*

- long interspersed elements (LINEs)*

- L1 family

- retrotransposons*

- ribosomal RNA genes

- **Few Functional Genes**

  - pseudogenes

- **Structural Variations**

  - copy number variations (CNVs)

  - Database of Genomic Variants (DGV)

Answers to Now Solve This

11.1 A circular chromosome, with no free ends present, avoids the problem faced by linear chromosomes, namely, complete replication of terminal sequences.

11.2 ^{3}H-thymidylic acid is a precursor of DNA. Because polytene chromosomes are formed by multiple rounds of DNA replication without strand separation, you would expect grains along the entire length of each polytene chromosome.

11.3 To perform volume calculations, assume the nucleus is a sphere and the chromosome is a cylinder.

Volume of the nucleus $= (4/3)\pi r^3$

$$= 4/3 \times 3.14 \times (5 \times 10^3 \text{ nm})^3$$
$$= 5.23 \times 10^{11} \text{ nm}^3$$

Volume of the chromosome $= \pi r^2 \times \text{length}$

$$= 3.14 \times (5.5 \text{nm})^2 \times (2 \times 10^9 \text{nm})$$
$$= 1.9 \times 10^{11} \text{ nm}^3$$

Therefore, the percentage of the volume of the nucleus occupied by the chromatin is

$$1.9 \times 10^{11} \text{nm}^3 / 5.23 \times 10^{11} \text{nm}^3 \times 100 = \text{about } 36.3\%$$

Solutions to Problems and Discussion Questions

1. (a) Higher-level circular chromosomal structures have been revealed through both chemical and observational (microscopic) analyses.

(b) Using radioactively labeled RNA precursors followed by autoradiography, researchers discovered a high rate of RNA incorporation, indicating intense transcription.

(c) Early evidence came from endonuclease digestion that yielded DNA fragments of about 200 base pairs in length. Electron microscopic, X-ray, and neutron-scattering observations revealed the structure of nucleosomes and their relationship to DNA.

(d) *In situ* hybridization studies show satellite DNA in clusters in heterochromatic regions that flank centromeres. In addition, base sequences and organizational motifs of satellite DNA are common to many regions within and flanking centromeric DNA. In humans, most satellite DNA is of the alphoid family found mainly in centromeric regions in tandem arrays of up to 1 million base pairs.

2. Your essay should include a description of overall chromosomal configuration (linear, circular, strandedness, etc.) as well as association with chromosomal proteins. In addition, it should describe higher-level structures, such as condensation in the case of eukaryotic chromosomes.

3. The bacteriophage λ chromosome is 17 μm in length. It exists as a linear, double-stranded DNA molecule while in the phage coat and closes to form a circular chromosome upon infection. T2 phage also has a linear, double-stranded DNA chromosome that is 52 μm long, about three times larger than that of λ phage. The *E. coli* chromosome, a circular, double-stranded molecule, is the largest of the three, having a length of about 1200 μm. Like bacterial chromosomes, the DNA of mitochondria and chloroplasts exists as double-stranded closed circles that replicate semiconservatively. Lengths of mtDNA but not cpDNA vary, and multiple copies of each DNA may occur in its respective organelle. They are both free of chromosomal proteins that are characteristic of eukaryotic chromosomes.

4. Polytene chromosomes appear in specific tissues (e.g., salivary glands) of many dipterans such as *Drosophila*. They are formed from numerous DNA replications and pairings of homologs in the absence of either strand separation or cytoplasmic division. Each chromosome contains about 1000 to 5000 DNA

strands in parallel register. They appear as comparatively long, wide fibers with sharp light and dark sections (bands) along their length. Such bands (chromomeres) are useful in chromosome identification and detection of chromosomal rearrangements.

5. Most puffs represent transcriptionally active genes, evidenced by staining and by the uptake of labeled RNA precursors, which can be assayed by autoradiography.

6. Lampbrush chromosomes are typically present in vertebrate oocytes and in spermatocytes of some insects. They are found during late prophase I and are active, uncoiled versions of condensed meiotic chromosomes.

7. Eukaryotes have a greater DNA content per cell than do bacteria and viruses, which may be due to the need for a variety of gene products in the many diverse cell types of multicellular eukaryotes. However, genomic size cannot be universally equated with an increase in complexity.

Seeing the question from a different perspective, it is likely that a much higher *percentage* of the genome of a bacterium is actually involved in phenotype production than in a eukaryote. Eukaryotes have obtained and maintain what appear to be large amounts of "extra" DNA. Bacteria, by contrast, are extremely efficient in their accumulation and use of their genome.

Given the larger amount of eukaryotic DNA per cell and the requirement that the DNA be partitioned in an orderly fashion to daughter cells during cell division, certain mechanisms and structures (mitosis, nucleosomes, centromeres, etc.) have evolved for packaging and distributing the DNA. In addition, the genome is divided into separate multiple chromosomes, perhaps to facilitate the partitioning processes in mitosis and meiosis.

8. X-ray diffraction studies of chromatin with and without histones suggested that histone-DNA interactions existed as regular, repeating structural units. This interpretation was supported by digestion of chromatin with micrococcal nuclease, which gave DNA fragments of approximately 200 base pairs or multiples of such segments. Further support came from observations of chromatin by electron microscopy that showed regularly spaced beadlike structures (nucleosomes). Kornberg's analysis of the interaction between histones and DNA led to his proposal that nucleosomes consisted of two types of histone tetramers associated with 200 bp of DNA. Further nuclease studies, in which digestion time was prolonged, revealed shortened DNA fragments (147 bp) and suggested the presence of linker DNA. Finally, neutron-scattering analysis of crystallized nucleosome core particles led to a detailed model of the nucleosome.

9. Nucleosomes are octameric structures of two molecules of each of the four core histones: H2A, H2B, H3, and H4. Each octamer consists of two tetramers—$(H2A)_2 \cdot (H2B)_2$ and $(H3)_2 \cdot (H4)_2$. Between the nucleosomes and complexed with linker DNA is histone H1. A 147-base-pair sequence of DNA wraps around the nucleosome in a left-handed helix that completes about 1.7 turns.

10. As chromosome condensation occurs, five or six nucleosomes coil together to form a 30 nm fiber called a solenoid. These fibers form a series of loops that further condense into the chromatin fiber, which is then coiled into chromosome arms making up each chromatid.

11. *Heterochromatin* is chromosomal material that stains deeply and remains condensed when other parts of chromosomes, euchromatin, are otherwise pale and less condensed. Heterochromatic regions replicate late in S phase and are relatively inactive in a genetic sense because there are few genes present or, if they are present, they are repressed. Telomeres and the areas adjacent to centromeres are composed of heterochromatin.

12. There are three main categories of repetitive sequences. (1) Satellite DNA is highly repetitive and consists of short, tandemly repeated sequences. It is found in heterochromatic regions of centromeres and telomeres. (2) Transposable sequences are varied in structure and size and are generally interspersed throughout the entire genome in eukaryotes.
(3) There are three types of middle repetitive tandem repeats, which vary in size and location. (i) Multiple-copy genes (such as rRNA genes) are large and are found at a single locus. (ii) Minisatellites (VNTRs), in which the repeated unit can be as long as 100 bp, are dispersed throughout the genome.
(iii) Microsatellites (STRs) are also dispersed throughout the genome, but the repeated sequence is only 2 to 5 bp in length.

13. Satellite DNA is identified by sedimentation equilibrium centrifugation as one or more additional peaks that represent DNA of a slightly different density than the majority (main band) of the genomic DNA. Satellite DNA falls into the highly repetitive category and consists of relatively large numbers of short sequences. Such sequences are clustered in heterochromatic areas typically flanking the centromere and in telomeres. Such areas are often void of typical euchromatic genes.

14. Both long interspersed elements (LINEs) and short interspersed elements (SINEs) are repetitive transposable DNA sequences in humans. SINEs are small, usually less than 500 bp, and are present in more than one million copies, whereas LINEs are quite large, usually 6 kb in length, and less prevalent (found about 850,000 times). LINEs are often referred to as retrotransposons because their mechanism of transposition (transcription to RNA, which is copied back to DNA by reverse transcriptase) resembles that used by retroviruses.

15. (a) Because there are 200 base pairs per nucleosome (as defined in this problem) and 10^9 base pairs, there would be 5×10^6 nucleosomes.

(b) Because there are 5×10^6 nucleosomes and nine histones (including H1) per nucleosome, there must be $9(5 \times 10^6) = 4.5 \times 10^7$ histone molecules.

(c) Because there are 10^9 base pairs present and each base pair is 0.34 nm, the overall length of the DNA is 3.4×10^8 nm. Dividing this value by the packing ratio (50) gives a compacted length of 6.8×10^6 nm.

16. The first step of this solution is to convert all of the given values to a common unit (e.g., μm or nm). Remember that 1 μm = 1,000 nm. Use the formulas $\pi r^2 h$ for the volume of a cylinder (DNA) and $(4/3)\pi r^3$ for the volume of a sphere (viral head).

Volume of DNA: $3.14 \times (1 \text{ nm})^2 \times (5 \times 10^4 \text{ nm}) =$

$$1.57 \times 10^5 \text{ nm}^3$$

Volume of capsid: $4/3 \times 3.14 \times (40 \text{ nm})^3 =$

$$2.68 \times 10^5 \text{ nm}^3$$

Because the capsid head has a greater volume than the volume of DNA, the DNA will fit into the capsid.

17. One base pair occupies 0.34 nm; therefore, the equation would be as follows:

52 μm/(0.34 nm/bp) × 1000 nm/μm =
$$152{,}941 \text{ base pairs}$$

18. Assuming a random distribution, dividing the size of the genome (3×10^9 base pairs) by the number of copies of the *Alu* element (10^6) gives, on average, one *Alu* sequence every 3000 base pairs. To be a little more precise, we might consider the size of the *Alu* sequences in our calculations. We know the approximate size of the *Alu* sequence to be 282 bp consensus sequence plus the A-rich region, so approximately 300 bp. Subtracting this value from the value calculated previously gives about 2700 bp between *Alu* sequences.

19. Bacteriophage lambda is composed of a double-stranded, linear DNA molecule of about 48,000 base pairs. It is capable of forming a closed, double-stranded circular molecule because of a 12-base-pair, single-stranded, complementary "overhanging" sequence at the 5' end of each single strand.

Chapter 12: The Genetic Code and Transcription

Concept Areas	Corresponding Problems
Genetic Code	1, 2, 8, 9, 12, 14, 15, 16, 23
Deciphering the Code	1, 3, 5, 6, 7, 9, 11, 12, 13, 15, 22, 23
Characteristics of the Code	1, 2, 3, 4, 5, 8, 9, 12, 13, 14, 15, 16, 22, 23
Information Flow	1, 2, 10, 13, 17, 18, 19, 23
RNA Structure	1, 11, 13, 20, 21, 24
RNA Processing	1, 20, 21, 24
Enzymology	10, 18, 19
Transcription	2, 17, 18, 19

Structures and Processes Checklist–Significant items that deserve special attention are identified with a "*".

(Check topic when mastered–provide examples where appropriate–understand the context of each entry)

- **Overview**
  - encoding of information
  - transfer of information
  - decoding of information
- **Genetic Code Characteristics***
  - linear
  - complementarity*
  - triplet code*
  - codon
  - unambiguous*
  - degenerate*
  - initiate*
  - terminate*
  - commaless
  - nonoverlapping
  - universal

- **Early Studies Established Code**
  - messenger RNA (mRNA)
  - frameshift mutations*
  - frame of reading*
- **Nirenberg, Matthaei, Others***
  - *in vitro* (cell-free) protein-synthesizing system*
  - polynucleotide phosphorylase*
  - no required template
  - RNA homopolymers*
  - RNA heteropolymers*
  - triplet frequency reflects nucleotide proportion in mix *
  - triplet binding assay*
  - transfer RNA (tRNA)
  - anticodon*
  - triplet RNA–ribosome complex

- o copolymers
- o repeating copolymers*
- o termination codons*
- o **Coding Dictionary***
  - o 61 amino acid assignments*
  - o three terminating triplets*
  - o pattern of degeneracy
  - o wobble hypothesis*
  - o 30 to 40 tRNA species*
  - o ordered genetic code
  - o N-formylmethionine (fMet)*
  - o initiator codon*
  - o methionine (eukaryotes)
  - o termination codons
  - o UAG, UAA, UGA*
  - o nonsense mutation*
- o **Genetic Code Confirmed***
  - o bacteriophage MS2
  - o colinearity*
  - o punctuation
- o **Nearly Universal Code***
  - o mtDNA*
  - o exceptions to the code
  - o shift in wobble base recognition
- o **Multiple Initiation Points**
  - o overlapping genes*
  - o limited amount of DNA
- o **Transcription of RNA from DNA***
  - o transcription*

- o information flow*
- o RNA as intermediate
- o **RNA Polymerase Directs RNA Synthesis**
  - o RNA polymerase*
  - o $n(\text{NTP}) \rightarrow (\text{NMP})_n + n(\text{PP}_i)$
  - o $(\text{NMP})_n + \text{NTP} \rightarrow (\text{NMP})_{n+1} + \text{PP}_i$
  - o core enzyme
  - o holoenzyme*
  - o sigma (σ) factor*
  - o template strand*
  - o coding strand*
  - o template binding
  - o promoters*
  - o transcription start site*
  - o consensus sequences*
  - o Pribnow box (-10 region), TATAAT *
  - o TTGACA (-35 region)
  - o *cis*-acting DNA elements*
  - o *trans*-acting factors*
  - o strong and weak promoters
  - o multiple forms of σ
  - o initiation
  - o chain elongation*
  - o 5'–3' extension*
  - o DNA/RNA duplex
  - o hairpin secondary structure
  - o intrinsic termination*
  - o rho-dependent termination*

- ○ termination factor, rho (ρ)
- ○ cistron*
- ○ polycistronic mRNA*
- ○ **Transcription in Eukaryotes***
  - ○ in nucleus
  - ○ three RNA polymerase forms
  - ○ chromatin remodeling*
  - ○ more DNA elements and protein factors
  - ○ complex termination
  - ○ RNA processing*
  - ○ pre-mRNA
  - ○ RNAP polymerase I (RNAP I)
  - ○ RNAP polymerase III (RNAP III)
  - ○ RNAP polymerase II (RNAP II)*
  - ○ core-promoter*
  - ○ proximal-promoter elements*
  - ○ enhancers*
  - ○ silencers*
  - ○ Goldberg–Hogness box, or TATA box*
  - ○ transcription factors
  - ○ general transcription factors (GTFs)*
  - ○ transcriptional activators
  - ○ transcriptional repressors
  - ○ TFIIA, TFIIB, TFIID, etc.
  - ○ pre-initiation complex
  - ○ polyadenylation signal sequence, AAUAAA*
  - ○ primary transcript

- ○ mature mRNA
- ○ posttranscriptional modification*
- ○ 7-methylguanosine (m^7G) cap*
- ○ 5′ to 5′ triphosphate bridge
- ○ poly-A polymerase*
- ○ poly-A tail*
- ○ poly-A binding protein*
- ○ **Coding Regions Interrupted***
  - ○ intervening sequence*
  - ○ intron*
  - ○ exon*
  - ○ RNA splicing*
  - ○ β-globin gene
  - ○ ovalbumin gene*
  - ○ *pro-α-2(1) collagen* gene
  - ○ alternative splicing*
  - ○ self-splicing RNAs
  - ○ ribozymes*
  - ○ transesterification reactions
  - ○ spliceosome*
  - ○ spliceosomal introns
  - ○ small nuclear RNAs (snRNAs)*
  - ○ small nuclear ribonucleoproteins (snRNPs)*
  - ○ donor sequence
  - ○ acceptor sequence
  - ○ branch point
  - ○ lariat

- **Modification of Final Transcript**
  - RNA editing
  - insertion/deletion editing*
  - substitution editing*
  - gRNA (guide RNA)*
  - glutamate receptor channels (GluR)

- **Transcription Visualized by Electron Microscopy**
  - *Xenopus laevis*
  - rDNA

Answers to Now Solve This

12.1 (a) The way to determine the fraction of each triplet that will occur with a random incorporation system is to determine the likelihood that each base will occur in each position of the codon (first, second, third), then multiply the individual probabilities (fractions) for a final probability (fraction), which can be converted to a percentage.

GGG	=	$3/4 \times 3/4 \times 3/4$	=	27/64 (42.2%)
GGC	=	$3/4 \times 3/4 \times 1/4$	=	9/64 (14.1%)
GCG	=	$3/4 \times 1/4 \times 3/4$	=	9/64 (14.1%)
CGG	=	$1/4 \times 3/4 \times 3/4$	=	9/64 (14.1%)
CCG	=	$1/4 \times 1/4 \times 3/4$	=	3/64 (4.7%)
CGC	=	$1/4 \times 3/4 \times 1/4$	=	3/64 (4.7%)
GCC	=	$3/4 \times 1/4 \times 1/4$	=	3/64 (4.7%)
CCC	=	$1/4 \times 1/4 \times 1/4$	=	1/64 (1.6%)

(b) Glycine:

GGG and one G_2C (adds up to 36/64 (56.2%)

Alanine:

one G_2C and one C_2G (adds up to 12/64 (18.8%)

Arginine:

one G_2C and one C_2G (adds up to 12/64 (18.8%)

Proline:

one C_2G and CCC (adds up to 4/64 (6.2%)

12.2 Assume that you have introduced a copolymer (ACACACAC...) to a cell-free protein-synthesizing system. There are two possibilities for establishing the reading frames: ACA if one starts at the first base and CAC if one starts at the second base. These would code for two different amino acids (ACA = threonine; CAC = histidine) and would produce repeating polypeptides that would alternate Thr-His-Thr-His... or His-Thr-His-Thr....

Because of a triplet code, a trinucleotide sequence will, once initiated, remain in the same reading frame and produce the same code all along the sequence regardless of the initiation site.

Given the sequence CUACUACUACUA, three different reading frames are defined, each of which produces a different sequence that contains a single amino acid:

Reading Frame: (1) CUA-CUA-CUA-CUA...

           Leu - Leu - Leu - Leu...

       (2) C - UAC-UAC-UAC-UAC...

           Tyr - Tyr - Tyr - Tyr ...

       (3) CU - ACU-ACU-ACU-ACU...

           Thr - Thr - Thr - Thr...

If a tetranucleotide is used, such as ACGUACGUACGU…, again there are three different reading frames, each of which produces a polypeptide that contains a repeating sequence of four amino acids. The sequences in all four polypeptides are the same (repeats of Thr-Tyr-Val-Arg) except that the starting amino acid changes.

Reading Frame: (1)   ACG-UAC-GUA-CGU-ACG-U…
                               Thr - Tyr - Val - Arg - Thr...

                       (2)   A - CGU-ACG-UAC-GUA-CGU...
                               Arg - Thr - Tyr - Val - Arg ...

                       (3)   AC - GUA-CGU-ACG-UAC-GUA...
                               Val - Arg - Thr - Tyr - Val...

12.3 (a) Apply complementary bases, substituting U for T:

Transcripts below are written in the 5′ to 3′ direction

     Sequence 1: 5′-AUGGCAAAAAAG-3′

     Sequence 2: 5′-AGUUAUUGAUGU-3′

     Sequence 3: 5′-AGAACCCUUGUA-3′

(b)   Sequence 1: Met-Ala-Lys-Lys

          Sequence 2: Ser-Tyr-(termination)

          Sequence 3: Arg-Thr-Leu-Val

(c) The coding strand has the same sequence as the mRNA, except T is substituted for U: 5′-ATGGCAAAAAAG-3′

Chapter 12 The Genetic Code and Transcription

Solutions to Problems and Discussion Questions

1. (a) Synthetic homopolymer and heteropolymer RNAs were created using polynucleotide phosphorylase. The frequencies of various nucleotide combinations (2 Gs and 1A, for example) were calculated from the relative abundance of each nucleotide in the reaction mixture. The synthetic RNAs were introduced into an *in vitro* translation system, and the amino acid compositions of the resulting polypeptides were determined. Comparison of relative frequencies of amino acids with the calculated frequencies of nucleotide combinations gave the base composition of codons, but not their actual sequence.

(b) The specific sequences of the triplet codes were initially determined by the triplet binding assay. These assignments were verified, and ambiguous results were clarified by *in vitro* translation of repeating copolymers of known sequence.

(c) Because the complete sequence of the RNA phage MS2 was known, scientists matched that sequence with protein products of MS2, which supported the code as derived from previous studies.

(d) Work with *E. coli* infected with phage showed that the synthesis of phage proteins appeared subsequent to and under the direction of newly synthesized RNA. Others were able to show that the newly synthesized RNA formed during a phage infection of bacteria would hybridize only with phage DNA, thus demonstrating the RNA to be the intermediary between phage DNA and protein.

(e) Primary transcripts were often noted to be longer than mature mRNAs, suggesting the loss of some sequences. The most direct evidence comes from direct comparison of the sequences of DNAs with their corresponding RNAs and proteins. Such studies show that DNA often contains sequences that are not represented in RNA and protein products.

2. Your essay should include a description of the nature and structure of the genetic code, the enzymes and logistics of transcription, and the chemical nature of RNA polymerization.

3. (a) Given a triplet code, the addition/loss of six nucleotides to a wild-type sequence will have no effect on the reading frame. The effect such an addition will have on an existing frameshift mutant will depend on the nature of the original mutation. If the frameshift were caused by addition of a single nucleotide, the reading frame could be restored by,

for example, the addition of two nucleotides or the loss of one. In other words, the translation system is "out of phase" until the third "+" or "–" is encountered.

(b) If the code were a sextuplet, then addition/loss only of six nucleotides would retain the reading frame in a wild-type sequence and the addition/loss of three or nine nucleotides would disrupt it. As for part (a) of this question, when nucleotides are added to an existing frameshift mutant, any addition or loss would need to compensate for the type of addition/loss that created the mutation.

4. The UUACUUACUUAC tetranucleotide sequence will produce the following triplets depending on the initiation point: UUA = Leu, UAC = Tyr, ACU = Thr, CUU = Leu. Notice that because of the degenerate code, two codons correspond to the amino acid leucine.

   The UAUCUAUCUAUC tetranucleotide sequence will produce the following triplets depending on the initiation point: UAU = Tyr, AUC = Ile, UCU = Ser, CUA = Leu. Notice that in this case, degeneracy is not revealed, and all the codons produce unique amino acids.

5. From the repeating polymer ACACA..., one can say that threonine is either CAC or ACA. From comparison of the polymer CAACAA... with ACACA..., ACA is the only codon in common. Therefore, threonine would have the codon ACA.

6. As in the previous problem, the procedure is to find those sequences that are the same for the first two bases but that vary in the third base. Given that AGG = Arg, information from the AG copolymer and understanding of the wobble hypothesis indicate that AGA also codes for Arg and GAG must therefore code for Glu.

   Coupling this information with that of the AAG copolymer, GAA must also code for Glu, and AAG must code for Lys.

7. In the assay, charged tRNAs are mixed with free ribosomes and many copies of a specific synthetic trinucleotide. If the trinucleotide is complementary to the anticodon of a charged tRNA, they will form a relatively large complex with the ribosome. This complex as well as free ribosomes are trapped on the filter due to their large size. By contrast, trinucleotides and charged tRNAs alone are small and will pass through the filter. If the amino acid on a charged, trapped tRNA is radioactive, then the filter becomes radioactive.

8. Make a table listing the original amino acids and the substitutions. Provide the codons for the original amino acids. Review the codons for the substituted amino acids, and select codons that provide single base changes. The base changes in the following examples are underlined.

Original		**Substitutions**
threonine	----->	alanine
<u>A</u>C (U, C, A, or G)		<u>G</u>C (U, C, A, or G)
glycine	----->	serine
<u>G</u>G (U or C)		<u>A</u>G (U or C)
isoleucine	----->	valine
<u>A</u>U (U, C or A)		<u>G</u>U (U, C or A)

9. Apply the most conservative pathway of change.

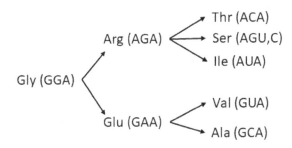

10. The enzyme generally functions in the degradation of RNA; however, in an *in vitro* environment, with high concentrations of the ribonucleoside diphosphates, the direction of the reaction can be forced toward polymerization. *In vivo*, the actual concentration of ribonucleoside diphosphates is low, so the degradative process is favored.

11. Because poly U is complementary to poly A, double-stranded structures will be formed. In order for an RNA to serve as a messenger RNA, it must be single-stranded, thereby exposing the bases for interaction with ribosomal subunits and tRNAs.

12. Applying the coding dictionary, the following sequences are "decoded":

Sequence 1: Met-Pro-Asp-Tyr-Ser-(term)

Sequence 2: Met-Pro-Asp-(term)

The 12th base (a uracil) is deleted from sequence 1, thereby causing a frameshift mutation that introduced a terminating triplet UAA.

13. **(a)** Below is one configuration that might occur with this particular sequence.

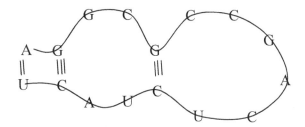

(b) 3′-TCCGCGGCTGAGATGA-5′ (use complementary bases, substituting T for U)

(c) 3′-GCU-5′

(d) Assuming that the AGG... is the first codon in the reading frame of the mRNA, the sequence would be

Arg-Arg-Arg-Leu-Tyr

14. Given the sequence GGA, by changing each of the bases to the remaining three bases and then checking the code table, one can determine whether amino acid substitutions will occur.

G G A Gly (wild-type)	G G U Gly (wild-type)
U G A **term**	U G U **Cys**
C G A **Arg**	C G U **Arg**
A G A **Arg**	A G U **Ser**
G U A **Val**	G U U **Val**
G C A **Ala**	G C U **Ala**
G A A **Glu**	G A U **Asp**
G G U Gly	G G A Gly
G G C Gly	G G C Gly
G G G Gly	G G G Gly

For both of these codons, changing the wobble base (three of the nine possible substitutions) will not result in an amino acid substitution. For the GGA codon, five of the remaining six single nucleotide substitutions result in an amino acid substitution at position 210. One results in premature translation termination. For the GGU codon, all six remaining single nucleotide substitutions result in an amino acid substitution.

15. (a) Starting from the 5' end and locating the AUG triplets, one finds two initiation sites leading to the following two sequences:

Met-His-Thr-Tyr-Glu-Thr-Leu-Gly

Met-Arg-Pro-Leu-(Asp or Glu)

(b) In the shorter of the two sequences (the one using the internal AUG triplet), the base substitution changed the second codon from an AGA triplet into a UGA triplet, and terminated the shorter product after the first amino acid. The remaining polypeptide is the longer one (the one using the first AUG codon), which has an amino acid substitution at residue five (from Glu to Val).

16. The number of codons for each particular amino acid (synonyms) is directly related to the frequency of amino acid incorporation stated in the problem. There are six codons for leucine, two for histidine, and only one for tryptophan.

17. Transcription describes the synthesis of RNA using a DNA template. The central dogma of molecular biology states that DNA produces, through transcription, RNA, much of which (mRNA) is "decoded" (during translation) to produce proteins. See F1.1 in Chapter 1 of this handbook for a graphic description.

18. RNA polymerase from *E. coli* is a large (almost 500,000 daltons) molecule composed of five subunit types (α, β, β', ω, and σ). The core enzyme contains four of these subunits, in the proportion of two copies of α, and single copies of each of β, β', and ω. The holoenzyme is the core with the addition of a dissociable subunit, σ. The β and β' subunits provide catalytic function, whereas the sigma (σ) subunit is responsible for the recognition of specific promoters.

19. Ribonucleoside triphosphates and a DNA template, in the presence of RNA polymerase and a divalent cation (Mg^{2+}), produce a ribonucleoside monophosphate polymer, DNA, and pyrophosphate. Equimolar amounts of precursor ribonucleoside triphosphates and products (ribonucleoside monophosphates and pyrophosphates) are formed. The polymer grows by sequential addition of ribonucleoside monophosphates, again, derived from ribonucleoside triphosphates, with the release of pyrophosphate.

20. Whereas some folding (from complementary base pairing) may occur with mRNA molecules, they generally exist as single-stranded structures, which are quite labile. Eukaryotic mRNAs are generally processed by the addition of a 5'-cap and a 3' poly-A tail. These features, which protect the eukaryotic mRNAs from degradation, are missing from bacterial messages, leaving them susceptible. Bacterial cells exist in a more unstable environment (nutritionally and physically, for example) as compared with that of eukaryotic cells; therefore, a rapid genetic response to environmental change is likely to be adaptive. To accomplish such rapid responses, a labile gene product (mRNA) is advantageous. A pancreatic cell, which is developmentally stable and exists in a relatively stable environment, could produce more insulin for a given transcriptional rate by using stable mRNAs.

21. It is likely that 3'-polyadenylation influences the overall conformation of RNA transcripts, which, in turn, affects the longevity of the transcript. One possible mechanism is the binding of proteins to the poly-A tail. In the case of eukaryotes, these proteins would be protective, whereas, in bacteria, degradative proteins would be recruited. In eukaryotes, 3'-polyadenylation might also influence the transport of RNAs to and from cellular organelles. In addition, 3'-polyadenylation might facilitate or inhibit the association of RNAs to other cellular components, such as proteins, lipids, or nucleic acids.

22. First, compute the frequency (percentages would be easiest to compare) for each of the random codons.

For 4/5 C: 1/5 A:

CCC = $4/5 \times 4/5 \times 4/5 = 64/125$ (51.2%)

C_2A = $3(4/5 \times 4/5 \times 1/5) = 48/125$ (38.4%)

CA_2 = $3(4/5 \times 1/5 \times 1/5) = 12/125$ (9.6%)

AAA = $1/5 \times 1/5 \times 1/5 = 1/125$ (0.8%)

For 4/5 A: 1/5 C:

AAA = $4/5 \times 4/5 \times 4/5 = 64/125$ (51.2%)

A_2C = $3(4/5 \times 4/5 \times 1/5) = 48/125$ (38.4%)

AC_2 = $3(4/5 \times 1/5 \times 1/5) = 12/125$ (9.6%)

CCC = $1/5 \times 1/5 \times 1/5 = 1/125$ (0.8%)

Proline:	C_3 and one of the C_2A triplets
Histidine:	one of the C_2A triplets
Threonine:	one C_2A triplet and one A_2C triplet
Glutamine:	one of the A_2C triplets
Asparagine:	one of the A_2C triplets
Lysine:	A_3

23. (a) Mutant 1: Nonsense mutation

Mutant 2: Missense mutation—a mutation that results in the replacement of one amino acid by another (see Chapter 14).

Mutant 3: Frameshift mutation

(b) Mutant 1: Mutation in the third position of the third triplet to A or G.

Mutant 2: Mutation in the first position of the third triplet from U to C.

Mutant 3: Removal of a G in the UGG (third) triplet (Trp).

(c) Termination

(d) All of the amino acids can be assigned specific triplets including the third base of each triplet. Compare the sequences for the wild type and mutant 3. After removal of a G in the UGG triplet of tryptophan, the frameshift mutation shifts the first base of the following triplet to the third (often ambiguous) base of the previous triplet. The only tricky solution is with serine, which has six triplet possibilities, but it can still be resolved.

AUG UGG UAU CGU GGU AGU CCA ACA

(e) The mutation may be in a promoter or enhancer, although many posttranscriptional alterations are possible.

24. (a) Alternative splicing occurs when copies of pre-mRNAs are spliced in more than one way, yielding various combinations of exons in the final mRNA products. Upon translation of a group of alternatively spliced mRNAs, a series of different, but related, proteins can be produced. The evolutionary advantage provided by alternative splicing is that an organism can encode more proteins without an increase in gene number. In other words, varieties of similar proteins can be produced by alternative splicing rather than by independent evolution.

(b) Some tissues might be more likely to develop alternative splicing if they depend on a number of related protein functions. In addition, alternative splicing can be used to generate varieties of slightly different products needed at different developmental stages.

Chapter 13: Translation and Proteins

<u>Concept Areas</u>	<u>Corresponding Problems</u>
Translation/Colinearity	2, 3, 4, 5, 6, 9, 15, 23
RNAs	1, 2, 3, 4, 5, 6, 7, 8, 14
Punctuation/Code	1, 13, 14, 15, 19
One-Gene:One-Enzyme	1, 10
Pathways	1, 20, 21, 22
Proteins	1, 2, 3, 11, 12, 13, 16, 17, 18
Ribosomes	2, 3, 14, 23

Structures and Processes Checklist–Significant items that deserve special attention are identified with a "*".

(Check topic when mastered–provide examples where appropriate–understand the context of each entry)

- **Overview**
  - information flow from RNA to polypeptides
  - protein structure and function
- **Translation of mRNA***
  - translation*
  - ribosomes*
  - transfer RNA (tRNA)*
  - adaptor hypothesis*
  - anticodon*
  - ribosome structure*
  - rRNA
  - ribosomal proteins
  - monosome
  - Svedberg coefficient (*S*)
  - 70S; 50S, 30S*
  - 80S; 60S, 40S*

- rDNA
- tandem repeats
- spacer DNA
- tRNA structure*
- cognate amino acid
- modified bases
- cloverleaf model of tRNA
- anticodon loop*
- ...pCpCpA-3′
- 5'-Gp...
- charging*
- aminoacyl tRNA synthetases*
- aminoacyladenylic acid
- isoaccepting tRNAs*
- **Steps in Translation***
  - initiation*
  - aminoacyl (A) site

- peptidyl (P) site
- exit (E) site
- initiation factors (IFs)
- N-formylmethionine (fMet)*
- Shine–Dalgarno sequence*
- initiation complex*
- elongation factors (EFs)
- elongation*
- peptidyl transferase*
- ribozyme*
- translocation
- termination*
- stop codons, termination codons, or nonsense codons
- release factors (RF1, RF2)
- polyribosomes, or polysomes*
- **High-Resolution Studies***
  - X-ray diffraction
  - platform
  - codon:anticodon accuracy check
  - time-resolved single particle cryo-electron microscopy (cryo-EM)
- **Translation in Eukaryotes***
  - core sequence
  - expansion sequences (ESs)
  - cap-dependent translation
  - eukaryotic initiation factors (eIFs)
  - scanning*
  - tRNA$_i^{Met}$*
  - Kozak sequence*

- poly-A binding proteins
- eIF4G
- eIF4E, or cap binding protein
- closed-loop translation*
- ribosome recycling*
- eukaryotic elongation factors (eEFs)
- eukaryotic release factors (eRFs)
- **Inborn Errors of Metabolism***
  - alkaptonuria*
  - alternative mode of metabolism
- **One-Gene:One-Enzyme**
  - *Neurospora* mutants*
  - one-gene:one-enzyme hypothesis*
  - complete medium
  - minimal medium
  - nutritional mutation*
- **Human Hemoglobin***
  - one-gene:one-protein hypothesis*
  - one-gene:one-polypeptide chain hypothesis*
  - sickle-cell anemia*
  - sickle-cell crisis
  - sickle-cell trait
  - HbA
  - HbS
  - inherited molecular disease*
- **Protein Structure***
  - polypeptides*
  - proteins*

- carboxyl group
- amino group
- R (radical) group*
- central carbon (C) atom
- nonpolar (hydrophobic)*
- polar (hydrophilic)*
- positively charged*
- negatively charged*
- peptide bond*
- dipeptide
- tripeptide
- primary structure*
- secondary structure*
- α-helix
- β-pleated sheet
- tertiary structure*
- quaternary structure*
- protein folding*
- thermodynamically stable conformation*
- chaperones*
- protein misfolding*
- ubiquitin*
- proteasome
- scrapie*
- bovine spongiform encephalopathy (mad cow disease)*

- Creutzfeldt–Jakob disease*
- prions*
- Huntington disease*
- Alzheimer disease*
- Parkinson disease*

- **Proteins and Diverse Functions***
  - hemoglobin
  - myoglobin
  - collagen
  - keratin
  - actin
  - myosin
  - tubulin
  - immunoglobulins
  - transport proteins
  - histones
  - transcription factors
  - enzymes
  - protein domains
  - catalytic domains
  - DNA-binding domains

F13.1 Polarity constraints associated with simultaneous transcription and translation in prokaryotes. The RNA polymerase is moving downward (arrow) in this sketch.

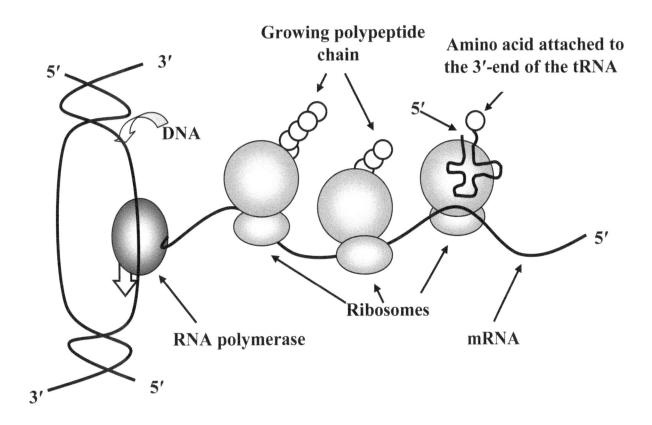

Answers to Now Solve This

13.1 One can conclude that the tRNA and not the amino acid is involved in recognition of the codon.

13.2 There are two codons for glutamic acid: GAA and GAG. With two of the codons for valine being GUA and GUG, a single base change in the second codon position of either (from A in glutamic acid to U in valine) could cause the Glu to Val switch. Likewise, a Glu to Lys switch could be caused by a single base change in the first codon position (from G in glutamic acid to A in lysine), converting either GAA to AAA or GAG to AAG. Glutamic acid (the amino acid normally present at position 6 of the β chain) is negatively charged, whereas valine is nonpolar and carries no net charge, and lysine is positively charged. Given these substantial charge changes, one would predict some, if not considerable, influence on protein structure and function. Such changes could stem from internal changes in folding (tertiary and/or quaternary structure) or interactions with other molecules in the RBC, especially other hemoglobin molecules.

Chapter 13 Translation and Proteins

Solutions to Problems and Discussion Questions

1. (a) The base sequences in tRNA suggested a cloverleaf secondary structure due to within-strand complementary base pairing. Such a model was later supported by X-ray crystallography and denaturation studies.

(b) In repeating copolymer experiments, polymers with unit sequences of either GAUA and GUAA directed incorporation of only a few amino acids (Chapter 12). This result was interpreted as showing the existence of termination codons. When UAA, UGA, or UAG triplets occur at internal sites in genes, premature translation termination occurs, which verifies the chain-terminating function of these triplets.

(c) Examination of nutritional mutations in *Neurospora* showed that upsets in metabolic pathways could result from mutant genes that segregated and assorted in typical fashion. In some cases, sufficient information was available to show that defective enzymes caused the metabolic upset. Thus, mutant genes must be responsible for the production of defective enzymes.

(d) Because enzymes (such as those in Beadle and Tatum's experiments) are proteins, it is reasonable to conclude that genes make proteins. In addition, early work on hemoglobin showed that one gene was responsible for making one of the polypeptide chains in hemoglobin.

2. Your essay should include descriptions of the ribosome and of translation, in which a functional ribosome, in conjunction with mRNA, orders amino acids and forms peptide bonds between them.

3. A functional polyribosome consists of many ribosomes bound to a single mRNA molecule. Each ribosome will contain the following components: mRNA, which carries the information from the DNA specifying the order of amino acids; a charged tRNA, which carries an amino acid into the ribosome; a large ribosomal subunit, which consists of proteins and rRNA, one of which (23S rRNA in bacteria) is responsible for the catalytic activity of the ribosome; a small ribosomal subunit, which consists of rRNA and proteins and which, in bacteria (via the 16S rRNA), is responsible for recognizing the translational start signal; perhaps initiation factors, which bind to the small ribosomal subunit to ensure proper interactions between the mRNA and the initiator tRNA; elongation factors, one of which escorts incoming charged tRNAs into the ribosome

and the other of which is responsible for ribosomal translocation; GTP, which provides the energy to release the amino acid from a charged tRNA as well as to induce a conformational change needed for translocation; Mg^{2+}; the growing polypeptide chain; and possibly release factors, which stimulate hydrolysis of the completed polypeptide from the peptidyl tRNA and dissociate the ribosomal subunits.

4. Transfer RNAs are "adaptor" molecules that provide a way for amino acids to interact with sequences of bases in nucleic acids. Amino acids are specifically and individually attached to the 3' end of tRNAs, which possess a three-base sequence (the anticodon) that can base-pair with three bases of mRNA (codons). Messenger RNA contains the instructions for the primary sequence of the peptide. It is a copy of the triplet codes that are stored in DNA. The sequences of bases in mRNA interact, three at a time, with the anticodons of tRNAs.

Enzymes involved in transcription include RNA polymerase (*E. coli*) or RNA polymerase I, II, III (eukaryotes). Those involved in translation include aminoacyl tRNA synthetases, the large subunit ribozyme, and release factors.

5. It was reasoned that there would not be sufficient affinity between amino acids and nucleic acids to account for protein synthesis. For example, acidic amino acids would not be attracted to nucleic acids. With an adaptor molecule, specific hydrogen bonding could occur between nucleic acids, and specific covalent bonding could occur between an amino acid and a nucleic acid tRNA.

6. The sequence of base triplets in mRNA constitutes the sequence of codons. A three-base portion of the tRNA constitutes the anticodon.

7. An amino acid in the presence of ATP, Mg^{2+}, and a specific aminoacyl synthetase produces an amino acid–AMP enzyme complex (+ PP_i). This complex interacts with a specific tRNA to produce the aminoacyl tRNA. See text Figure 13.5.

8. The four sites in tRNA that provide for specific recognition are sites for attachment of the specific amino acid; interaction with the aminoacyl tRNA synthetase; interaction with the ribosome; and interaction with the codon (anticodon).

9. There are many key differences between translation in bacteria and translation in eukaryotes, nine of which are described below:

1) *Coupling of transcription and translation*: Coupling can occur in bacteria because both processes take place in the cytoplasm but is not possible in eukaryotes because the two processes are spatially separated (nucleus vs. cytoplasm)

2) *Ribosome size and composition*: Eukaryotic ribosomes are larger than those in bacteria, consisting of more proteins and larger rRNA molecules. Although bacterial and eukaryotic rRNAs share core sequences, eukaryotic rRNAs also contain expansion segments. In addition, the large ribosomal subunit of eukaryotes also contains an additional form of rRNA.

3) *Mechanism of ribosome binding*: In bacteria, initiation depends on base-pairing interactions between the small subunit 16S rRNA and the Shine–Dalgarno sequence of the message. By contrast, in eukaryotes, translation is cap-dependent, in which the small ribosomal subunit associates with the 5′-m^{7}G cap.

4) *Initiation factors*: Bacteria use three initiation factors, whereas eukaryotes require a suite of initiation factors.

5) *Mechanism of identifying the translational start*: In bacteria, an initiation factor (IF2) binds to both the charged initiator tRNA and the mRNA start codon, and stabilizes them in the P site. In eukaryotes, after the small subunit, the charged initiator tRNA and several initiation factors have assembled at the 5′-cap, the assembly slides along the message, scanning for the Kozak consensus sequence, which contains the start site.

6) *Identity of the first amino acid*: Although both bacteria and eukaryotes use a special initiator charged tRNA and both incorporate methionine as the first amino acid, bacteria incorporate a chemically modified form of methionine (N-formylmethionine).

7) *Linear vs. closed-loop translation*: The 5′- and 3′-ends of bacterial messages do not interact; therefore, ribosomes traverse the molecule from one end to the other. In eukaryotes, however, poly-A binding proteins interact with several initiation factors, linking the 5′- and 3′-ends. Closed-loop translation allows for eukaryotic ribosome recycling.

8) *Message stability*: Due to their 5′-caps and 3′-poly-A tails, eukaryotic messages are more stable than those in bacteria. This means that eukaryotic messages are available to be translated for a longer period of time.

9) *Release factors*: Bacteria use three release factors, whereas eukaryotes use only one.

10. Given that enzymes are one subclass of *proteins*, a more general statement of *one-gene:one-protein* might seem to be more appropriate. However, some proteins are made up of subunits, with each different type of subunit (polypeptide chain) being under the control of a different gene. Under this circumstance, the statement *one-gene:one-polypeptide* might be more reasonable.

It turns out that many functions of cells and organisms are controlled by stretches of DNA that either produce no protein product (operator and promoter regions, for example) or have more than one function (overlapping genes and alternative splicing of mRNA). A simple statement regarding the relationship of a stretch of DNA to its physical product is difficult to justify.

11. The quaternary level, which results from the associations of individual polypeptide chains.

12. Sickle-cell anemia is coined a *molecular* disease because it is well understood at the molecular level; there is a base change in DNA, which leads to an amino acid change in the β chain of hemoglobin. It is considered to be a *genetic* disease because it is inherited from one generation to the next. Sickle-cell anemia is not contagious, unlike many diseases caused by microorganisms. Furthermore, infectious diseases would not necessarily follow family pedigrees, whereas genetic diseases do. Finally, infectious diseases can often be cured, whereas inherited diseases cannot.

13. A person who has the sickle-cell allele in the heterozygous state is a carrier. A person who is homozygous for the sickle-cell allele has sickle-cell anemia. In the sickle-cell allele, a single base change occurs in the DNA that encodes the sixth amino acid position in the β chain of hemoglobin, which causes the incorporation of valine instead of glutamic acid. As a result, both the structure and function of the hemoglobin molecule are altered.

14. Given that each nucleotide is 0.34 nm long, we can calculate that each triplet is about 1 nm in length. If the diameter of a ribosome is 20 nm, approximately 20 codons could be found in that ribosome.

15. The wild-type and mutant alleles of the gene encoding the T4 head protein could be isolated and sequenced and the sequences compared. Likewise, the amino acid sequences of both wild-type and mutant forms of the head protein could also be compared. Having the precise intragenic location of mutations as well as the locations of the premature termination points in the mutant phage proteins, colinearity can be examined.

If genes and their protein products are colinear, the location of mutations should correspond with the sites of early termination. In this problem, therefore, the nearer the mutations to the 5' end of the mRNA, the shorter the polypeptide product.

16. As stated in the text, the four levels of protein structure are the following:

Primary: the linear arrangement or sequence of amino acids. This sequence ultimately determines the higher-level structures.

Secondary: the folding of the peptide backbone that results in repeating structures (such as the α-helix and β-pleated sheet), which are stabilized by hydrogen bonds between components of the peptide bond.

Tertiary: three-dimensional folding that occurs as a result of interactions among the amino acid side chains. These interactions include, but are not limited to, the following: covalent disulfide bonds between cysteine residues, interactions of hydrophilic side chains with water, and interactions of hydrophobic side chains with each other.

Quaternary: the association of two (dimer) or more polypeptide chains.

Because all higher levels are dependent on the sequence of amino acids (primary structure), it is the primary structure that is most influential in determining protein structure and function.

17. There are probably as many different types of proteins as there are different types of structures and functions in living systems. Some examples follow:

Oxygen transport: hemoglobin, myoglobin
Structural: collagen, keratin, histones
Contractile: actin, myosin
Immune system: immunoglobulins
Cross-membrane transport: a variety of proteins in and around membranes, such as receptor proteins

Regulatory: hormones, perhaps histones

18. Enzymes function to regulate the catabolic and anabolic activities of cells. They lower the *energy of activation,* thus allowing chemical reactions to occur under conditions (e.g., temperature, pH) that are compatible with living systems. Enzymes possess active sites and/or other domains that are sensitive to the environment. The active site is considered to be a crevice, or pit, that binds reactants, thus enhancing their interaction. The other domains mentioned above may influence the conformation and therefore the function of the active site.

19. All of the substitutions involve one base change.

20. Even though three gene pairs are involved, notice that because of the pattern of mutations, each cross may be treated as monohybrid **(a)** or dihybrid **(b, c)**.

(a) F_1: $AABbCC$ = speckled

F_2: 3 $AAB-CC$ = speckled
  1 $AAbbCC$ = yellow

(b) F_1: $AABbCc$ = speckled

F_2: 9 $AAB-C-$ = speckled
  3 $AAB-cc$ = green
  3 $AAbbC-$ = yellow ⎱
  1 $AAbbcc$ = yellow ⎰ 4

(c) F_1: $AaBBCc$ = speckled

F_2: 9 $A-BBC-$ = speckled
  3 $A-BBcc$ = green
  3 $aaBBC-$ = colorless ⎱ 4
  1 $aaBBcc$ = colorless ⎰

21. Because cross **(a)** is essentially a monohybrid cross, there would be no difference in the results if crossing over occurred (or did not occur) between the *A* and *B* loci.

22. The best way to approach these types of problems, especially when the data are organized in the form given, is to realize that the substance (supplement) that "repairs" or "rescues" a strain, as indicated by a (+), is *after* the metabolic block for that strain. In addition, and most important, the substance that rescues the highest number of strains either is *the end product* or is *closest to the end product.*

The data in the table indicate that the supplement tryptophan (TRP) rescues all the strains. Therefore, it must be at the end of the pathway or at least after all of the metabolic blocks (defined by each mutation). Indole (I) rescues the next highest number of strains (3); therefore, it must be second from the end. Indole glycerol phosphate (IGP) repairs two of the four strains, so it is third from the end. Anthranilic acid (AA) repairs the least number of strains, so it must be early (first) in the pathway.

Minimal medium is void of supplements: Mutant strains involving this pathway would not be expected to grow (or be rescued) by this medium. The pathway therefore would be as follows:

AA----->IGP----->I----->TRP

To assign the various mutations to the pathway, keep in mind that if a supplement rescues a given mutant, the supplement must be after the metabolic block. Applying this rationale to the pathway, the metabolic blocks are created at the following locations:

trp-8   trp-2   trp-3 trp-1

precursor-->AA--->IGP-->I-->TRP

23.

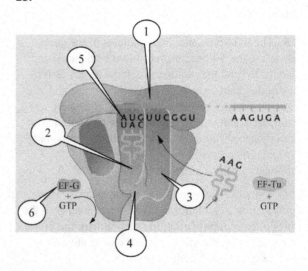

Chapter 14: Gene Mutation, DNA Repair, and Transposition

Concept Areas	Corresponding Problems
Classes of Mutations	1, 3, 4, 7, 8, 11, 15, 25
Detection of Mutations	1, 2, 4, 7, 16, 21, 23
Spontaneous Mutation Rates	3, 21
Molecular Basis of Mutation	2, 7, 8, 9, 10, 11, 12, 15, 19, 22, 23, 25
Repair of DNA	1, 2, 13, 17, 22, 23
UV Radiation and Skin Cancer	17, 23
High-Energy Radiation	12, 14
Transposable Elements	18, 19, 20, 24
Case Studies, Human Impact	14, 15, 17, 22, 23
Cellular Responses to Mutations	2, 4, 5, 6, 11, 16, 17, 25
Mutagens/Carcinogens	1, 10, 12, 14, 16

Structures and Processes Checklist–Significant items that deserve special attention are identified with a "*".

(Check topic when mastered–provide examples where appropriate–understand the context of each entry)

- **Overview**
  - gene mutations
- **Classification of Gene Mutations***
  - alteration in nucleotide sequence
  - type of molecular change*
  - point mutation, or base substitution*
  - missense mutation*
  - nonsense mutation*
  - silent mutation*
  - neutral mutation*
  - transition
  - transversion
  - frameshift mutation*
  - effect on function*
- loss-of-function mutation*
- null mutations*
- recessive mutation
- dominant mutation
- dominant negative mutation*
- haploinsufficiency
- gain-of-function mutation*
- suppressor mutation
- intragenic mutation
- intergenic mutation
- location of mutation*
- somatic mutation*
- autosomal mutation
- X-linked mutation
- Y-linked mutation

- mutations in germ line
- homogametic sex
- hemizygous

- **Mutations are Spontaneous or Induced**
  - spontaneous mutation
  - induced mutation
  - mutation rate*
  - mutation hot spots
  - single-nucleotide polymorphisms (SNPs)

- **Replication Errors and Base Modifications***
  - misincorporated nucleotides
  - tautomers*
  - replication slippage
  - tautomeric shifts*
  - depurination*
  - apurinic site
  - deamination*
  - oxidative damage
  - reactive oxidants*

- **Induced Mutations***
  - mutagen*
  - base analogs*
  - 5-bromouracil (5-BU)
  - bromodeoxyuridine (BrdU)
  - alkylating agents
  - ethyl methanesulfonate (EMS)
  - intercalating agents

- adduct-forming agents
- electromagnetic spectrum
- ultraviolet (UV) radiation*
- pyrimidine dimers*
- X rays
- gamma rays
- cosmic rays
- ionizing radiation*
- free radicals*

- **Single-Gene Mutations***
  - polygenic*
  - monogenic*
  - single nucleotide changes
  - promoter mutations*
  - splicing mutations*
  - β-thalassemia
  - β-globin (*HBB*) gene

- **DNA Repair Systems***
  - DNA repair
  - DNA polymerase III*
  - proofreading*
  - mismatch repair (MMR)*
  - endonuclease*
  - exonuclease*
  - postreplication repair*
  - homologous recombination repair
  - SOS repair system*
  - photoreactivation repair*
  - UV-induced DNA damage*

- ○ photoreactivation enzyme (PRE)*
- ○ photolyase
- ○ excision repair*
- ○ base excision repair (BER)*
- ○ DNA glycosylase*
- ○ apyrimidinic site*
- ○ apurinic site*
- ○ AP endonuclease*
- ○ nucleotide excision repair (NER)*
- ○ xeroderma pigmentosum (XP)*
- ○ UV-induced lesions
- ○ somatic cell hybridization*
- ○ heterokaryon*
- ○ complementation*
- ○ *DNA polymerase eta (POLH)* gene*
- ○ double-stranded break (DSB) repair*
- ○ homologous recombination repair*
- ○ nonhomologous end joining

- ○ **Assessing Mutagenicity***
  - ○ Ames test*
  - ○ *Salmonella typhimurium*
  - ○ *his⁺* revertants*
  - ○ metabolic activation*
  - ○ carcinogens

- ○ **Mobile DNA Elements***
  - ○ transposable elements (TEs)*
  - ○ DNA transposons*
  - ○ inverted terminal repeats (ITRs)
  - ○ transposase*
  - ○ direct repeats (DRs)
  - ○ autonomous transposons
  - ○ nonautonomous transposons
  - ○ "cut-and-paste" mechanism
  - ○ Ac-Ds system*
  - ○ *Dissociation (Ds)*
  - ○ *Activator (Ac)*
  - ○ mobile controlling element*
  - ○ retrotransposons
  - ○ RNA intermediate
  - ○ "copy-and-paste" mechanism
  - ○ reverse transcriptase
  - ○ integrase
  - ○ *copia**
  - ○ long terminal repeat (LTR)
  - ○ *white-apricot* mutation
  - ○ long interspersed elements (LINEs)*
  - ○ short interspersed elements (SINEs)*
  - ○ insertions into human genes
  - ○ *Alu* element*
  - ○ evolutionary implications*

F14.1 Graphic representation of the relationship between mutation and Darwinian evolutionary theory. Mutation provides the original source of variation on which natural selection operates.

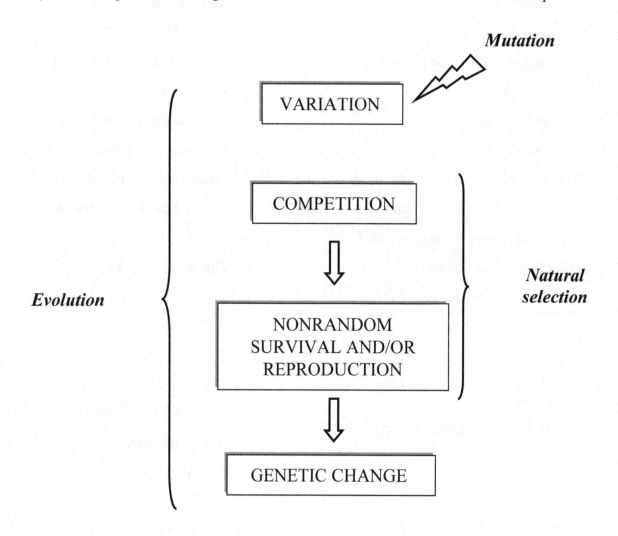

F14.2 Illustration of the difference between somatic and germ-line mutations. Somatic mutations are not passed to the next generation, whereas those in the germ line might be passed to offspring.

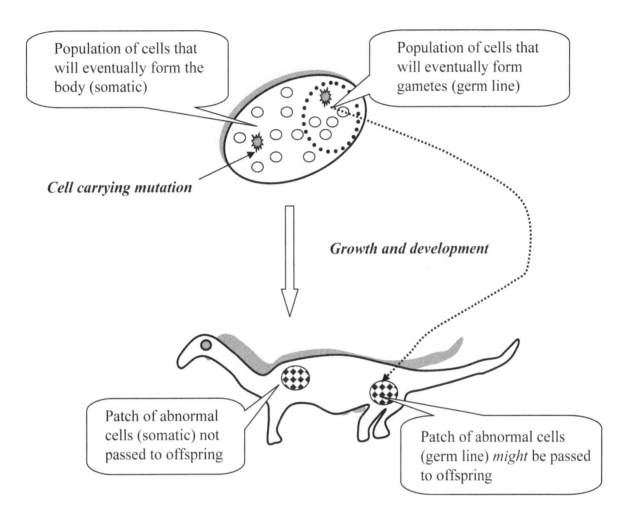

Chapter 14 Gene Mutation, DNA Repair, and Transposition

Answers to Now Solve This

14.1 The phenotypic influence of any base change is dependent on a number of factors, including its location in coding or noncoding regions, its potential in dominance or recessiveness, and its interaction with other base sequences in the genome. If a base change is located in a noncoding region, there may be no influence on the phenotype; however, some noncoding regions serve regulatory functions—mutations that influence transcription levels, poly-A addition, splicing, and translation could affect phenotype. If a mutation occurring in a coding region acts as a full recessive, there should be no influence on the phenotype; however, if the mutant allele acts as a dominant, then there would be an influence on the phenotype. Some genes interact with other genes in a variety of ways that would be difficult to predict without additional information.

14.2 There are several ways in which an unexpected mutant allele may enter a pedigree. If an allele is incompletely penetrant, it may be present in a population and only express itself under certain conditions. It is unlikely that the allele for hemophilia behaved in this manner. If a gene's expression is suppressed by another mutation in an individual, it is possible that offspring may inherit that given gene and not inherit its suppressor. Such offspring would have hemophilia. Because all genetic variations must arise at some point, it is possible that the mutation in Queen Victoria's family was a new germ-line mutation, arising in her father. Last, it is possible (but not very probable) that her mother was heterozygous and, by chance, no other individuals in her mother's family received the mutant allele.

14.3 Any agent that inhibits DNA replication, either directly or indirectly, through mutation and/or DNA crosslinking, will suppress the cell cycle and might be useful in cancer therapy. Guanine alkylation often leads to mismatched bases, which can often be repaired by a variety of repair mechanisms. DNA cross linking can be repaired as well, using recombinational mechanisms. Thus, for such agents to be successful in cancer therapy, suppressors of DNA repair systems are often used in conjunction with certain cancer drugs. See Wang, Z. et al. 2001. J Nat'l Cancer Inst. 93(19):1434–6.

14.4 Ethyl methanesulfonate (EMS) alkylates the keto groups at the sixth position of guanine and at the fourth position of thymine. In each case, base-pairing affinities are altered and transition mutations result. Altered bases are not readily repaired if mismatch repair systems are nonfunctional, and once the transition to normal bases occurs through replication, such mutations avoid repair altogether.

Chapter 14 Gene Mutation, DNA Repair, and Transposition
Solutions to Problems and Discussion Questions

1. (a) The Ames test assesses mutagenicity of compounds by testing their ability to cause *his⁻* strains of *Salmonella typhimurium* to revert to *his⁺*. When known carcinogens were tested, more than 80 percent were found to also be potent mutagens

(b) Various chemicals and radiation have been tested by a number of screening strategies, such as the Ames test, described in 1(a), or assessment of phenotypic change in a model organism after exposure to a potential mutagen. When the frequency of mutation in a test organism increases in concert with exposure to a given agent, that agent is classified as a mutagen.

(c) In addition to postreplication repair, SOS, photo-reactivation, and excision repair, various proofreading functions have been discovered in polymerases. Each has provided evidence that many mutations, once generated, may trigger repair. The correlation between mutation of the genes whose products control DNA repair and the observation of genome hypermutability, human DNA repair diseases, and cancers supports the conclusion that these systems successfully correct the majority of mutations.

2. Your essay should include a brief description of the genomic differences between eukaryotes and bacteria and the ways that ploidy influences the phenotypic effects of mutations in one copy of a gene. You should also include a summary of repair pathways that operate predominantly in bacteria or predominantly in eukaryotes, as well as a description of the differences in repair pathways that are shared by both types of organisms.

3. Mutations that occur as a result of natural biological and/or chemical processes are considered spontaneous. They are relatively rare in comparison to induced mutations, which result from the action of external agents and tend to cause physical or chemical damage to DNA.

4. The extent to which a mutation changes the characteristics of an organism depends on the type of mutation (dominant or recessive), the type of cell affected (proliferating or nonproliferating), the number of cells affected, and the degree to which the mutation alters the function of the gene product or regulatory region. A recessive somatic mutation would not produce a visible phenotype in a diploid organism. A dominant mutation would be more likely to be visible if it occurs early in development. However, if only a relatively small number of cells are affected, the effects of a dominant mutation could be masked by surrounding nonmutant cells. Similarly, if the mutation does not cause substantial alterations to the gene product or to regulation of expression of this product, an effect may not be visible. Mutations that occur in somatic cells are not transmitted to the next generation but may lead to altered cellular function or tumors.

5. It is true that *most* mutations are thought to be deleterious to an organism. A gene is a product of perhaps a billion or so years of evolution, and it is only natural to suspect that random changes will probably yield negative results. However, mutations create the variation for natural selection to work with, and *all* mutations may not be deleterious. Those few, rare variations that are beneficial will provide a basis for possible differential propagation of the variation. Such changes in gene frequency represent the basis of the evolutionary process. See F14.1 in this handbook.

6. As stated in the previous answer, a functional sequence of nucleotides, a gene, is likely to be the product of perhaps a billion or so years of evolution honed by natural selection to an optimal state for a given environment, components of which have also evolved, or coevolved. Deviations from the norm, caused by mutation, are likely to be disruptive because of the complex and interactive environment in which each gene product must function. However, on occasion a beneficial variation occurs.

7. A diploid organism possesses at least two copies of each gene (except for "hemizygous" genes), and in most cases, the amount of product from one copy of each pair is sufficient for production of a normal phenotype. Recall that the condition of "recessive" is defined by the phenotype of the heterozygote. If output from one normal (nonmutant) gene in a heterozygote gives the same phenotype as in the normal homozygote (where there are two normal copies), the normal allele is considered "dominant."

	Phenotype, if mutant allele is	
Genotype	**recessive**	**dominant**
wild/wild	wild	wild
wild/mutant	wild	mutant
mutant/mutant	mutant	mutant

8. A silent mutation is a point mutation in an open reading frame that does not alter the amino acid encoded, due to degeneracy of the genetic code. A neutral mutation is one that occurs in noncoding DNA and does not affect gene products or gene expression.

9. Watson and Crick recognized that various tautomeric forms, which are caused by single proton shifts, could exist for the nitrogenous bases of DNA. Such shifts could result in mutations by allowing hydrogen bonding between bases that are usually noncomplementary. As stated in the text, biologically important tautomers involve keto–enol pairs for thymine and guanine and amino–imino pairs for cytosine and adenine. Replication of the strand containing the anomalous base will result in a point mutation.

10. All three agents are mutagenic because they cause base substitutions, specifically transitions, but by different mechanisms. Deaminating agents oxidatively convert an amino group to a keto group such that cytosine is converted to uracil and pairs with adenine while adenine is converted to hypoxanthine and pairs with cytosine. Alkylating agents donate an alkyl group to the amino or keto groups of nucleotides, thus altering base-pairing affinities. 6-ethyl guanine acts like adenine, thus pairing with thymine. Base analogs such as 5-bromouracil and 2-amino purine are incorporated as thymine and adenine, respectively, yet they base-pair with guanine and cytosine, respectively.

11. Frameshift mutations are likely to change more than one amino acid in a protein product because as the reading frame is shifted, a different set of codons is generated. In addition, there is the possibility that a nonsense triplet could be introduced, thus causing premature chain termination. If a single pyrimidine or purine has been substituted, then only one amino acid is influenced.

12. X rays are of higher energy and shorter wavelength than UV light. They have greater penetrating ability and can create more disruption of DNA.

13. *Photoreactivation* can lead to repair of UV-induced damage. An enzyme, photoreactivation enzyme, will absorb a photon of light to cleave thymine dimers. *Excision repair* involves the products of several genes plus DNA polymerase I and DNA ligase, to clip out the UV-induced dimer, fill in the resulting gap, and join the phosphodiester backbone. The excision repair process can be activated by damage that distorts the DNA helix. *Recombinational repair* is a postreplication repair system that responds to DNA that escaped repair at the time of replication. If a gap is created when DNA polymerase stalls and skips replication on one of the newly synthesized strands, recombinational repair fills this gap by allowing genetic exchange with the undamaged template strand of the same polarity. The resulting gap on the donor strand is filled by repair synthesis. The *SOS repair system* is activated when numerous mismatches and gaps are detected. Random or incorrect nucleotides are often incorporated at sites where DNA polymerase would normally stall; therefore, this is called an "error-prone system."

14. Because mammography involves the use of X rays, which are known to be mutagenic, it has been suggested that frequent mammograms may do harm. This subject is presently under considerable debate. Although data show that screening decreases overall mortality from breast cancer, the side effects of exposure to diagnostic radiation are often difficult to identify and quantify.

15. Many mutations in regions upstream from coding regions in a gene alter sequences recognized by transcription factors and/or polymerase and thereby influence transcription. Mutations within introns may affect intron splicing or other factors that determine mRNA stability or translation.

16. In the *Ames assay,* the compound to be tested is incubated with a mammalian liver extract to simulate an *in vivo* environment. This solution is then placed on culture plates with an indicator microorganism, *Salmonella typhimurium,* which is defective in its normal repair processes as well as being unable to synthesize histidine. The frequency of his^+ revertants in the tester strains is an indication of the mutagenicity of the compound. Because cancers arise through mutation, it makes sense to think that mutagens are potential carcinogens. In the 1970s, more than 80 percent of carcinogens tested by this method were shown to be mutagenic.

17. *Xeroderma pigmentosum* is a rare recessive disorder in which affected individuals are highly sensitive to UV radiation and have a 2000-fold higher incidence of cancer than unaffected individuals. Cells from XP patients are defective in the nucleotide excision repair (NER) system, which recognizes and corrects "bulky" lesions in DNA, such as pyrimidine dimers. Studies with heterokaryons provided evidence for at least seven different genes involved in the NER pathway. Because cancer is caused by mutations in several types of genes, interfering with DNA repair can enhance the occurrence of these types of mutations. Phenotypes of XP include extreme sensitivity to UV light and skin cancer. UV irradiation causes thymidine dimers, which go undetected in the absence of a functional NER pathway. Because cancer is caused by mutations in several types of genes, interfering with DNA repair can enhance the occurrence of these types of mutations.

18. Both DNA transposons and retrotransposons are able to move from one DNA location to another and both can be either autonomous (able to synthesize their own transposase) or nonautonomous. Most DNA transposons move using a "cut-and-paste" mechanism that removes it from one location and inserts it into another site. A retrotransposon, by contrast, uses a "copy-and-paste" mechanism of transfer. An RNA intermediate is transcribed and converted into double-stranded DNA, which is inserted back into the genome by integrase. Retrotransposons are not removed from the original integration site.

19. In some cases, chromosome breakage occurs that has significant influence on gene function. In other cases, deletions may occur, which also influence gene function.

20. By insertion into the transcriptional regulatory region of a gene, a transposon could cause the gene to be expressed at a different developmental time or under different circumstances, due to the presence of the TE's own promotor or enhancers. Alternatively, the presence of multiple copies of a transposon in the genome could result in recombination between copies on different chromosomes, leading to chromosomal rearrangements. In most cases, changes in DNA are harmful to organisms, whereas in rare cases, an evolutionary advantage occurs because the new genetic variation confers a selective advantage.

21. Given that the cells were treated and then allowed to complete one round of replication, the final computation of the mutation rate should be divided by two (two cells are plated for each cell treated). The general expression for the mutation rate is the number of mutant cells divided by the total number of cells. In this case, the equation is as follows:

$$\frac{18 \times 10^1}{6 \times 10^7}$$

or 3×10^{-6}

Dividing by two (as stated above) gives

$$1.5 \times 10^{-6}$$

22. Unscheduled DNA synthesis represents DNA repair. Strains that do not complement one another in a heterokaryon (indicated by a "−") are defective in the same gene and, therefore, are in the same complementation group. Strains that do show complementation (indicated by a "+") have mutations in different genes and are in different complementation groups. For instance, *XP1* and *XP2* are placed into the same complementation group, but *XP1* and *XP5* are in different groups. Analysis of all the data gives the following groupings:

Group 1: *XP1, XP2, XP3*

Group 2: *XP4*

Group 3: *XP5, XP6, XP7*

The complementation groups indicate that there are at least three genes that form products necessary for unscheduled DNA synthesis. All of the cell lines that are in the same complementation group are defective in the same product.

23. (a) Individuals with xeroderma pigmentosum (XP) are much more likely than non-XP individuals to contract skin cancer in youth. By age 20, approximately 80 percent of the XP population has skin cancer compared with approximately 4 percent in the non-XP group.

(b) XP individuals lack one or more functional genes involved in DNA repair.

24. First, although less likely, one might suggest that transposons are more likely to insert in noncoding regions of the genome. One might also suggest that they are more stable in such regions. Second, and more likely, it is possible that transposons insert randomly and that selection eliminates those that have interrupted coding regions of the genome. Because such regions are more likely to influence the phenotype, selection is more likely to influence such regions.

25. **(a)** Nonsense mutation in coding regions: The product will be shorter than 375 amino acids. The final size will depend on where the chain termination occurred.

(b) Insertion in exon 1, causing frameshift: a variety of amino acid substitutions and possible premature chain termination downstream.

(c) Insertion in exon 7, causing frameshift: a variety of amino acid substitutions and possible premature chain termination downstream. Only the final two exons will be affected, as opposed to the product created by the insertion in exon 1.

(d) Missense mutation: a single change in which one amino acid is substituted for another. The remainder of the protein is unchanged.

(e) Deletion in exon 2, causing frameshift: amino acids will be missing; the actual number will depend on the size of the deletion. The frameshift would cause additional amino acid changes and possible premature chain termination.

(f) Deletion in exon 2, in frame: amino acids missing from exon 2 without additional changes in the protein.

(g) Large deletion covering Exons 2 and 3: significant loss of amino acids toward the N-terminal side of the protein.

Chapter 15: Regulation of Gene Expression in Bacteria

Concept Areas	Corresponding Problems
Overview of Bacterial Gene Regulation	1, 2, 3, 4
Lactose Metabolism in E. coli	1, 5, 6, 7, 10, 13
Inducible and Repressible Systems	1, 2, 4, 5, 6, 10, 11, 14
Repressor Molecules	1, 4, 7, 8, 9
Positive and Negative Control	2, 3, 10, 14
Catabolite Repression	10
Tryptophan Operon	1, 12, 13
Model Systems	11, 14
Attenuation	12, 13
Regulation by RNA	12, 13, 15
CRISPR-Cas	16, 17, 18

Structures and Processes Checklist—Significant items that deserve special attention are identified with a "*".

(Check topic when mastered–provide examples where appropriate–understand the context of each entry)

- **Overview**
  - responsive to environmental conditions
  - responsive to phage infection
- **Bacterial Gene Regulation***
  - metabolic needs
  - inducible enzymes*
  - constitutive enzymes*
  - repressible*
  - negative control*
  - positive control*
  - regulator molecule
- **Lactose Metabolism in *E. coli***
  - inducer*
  - operon*

- regulatory region
- *cis*-acting site*
- *trans*-acting factors*
- lactose (*lac*) operon
- structural genes
- *lacZ* gene
- *β*–galactosidase*
- *lacY* gene
- permease*
- *lacA* gene
- transacetylase
- polycistronic mRNA
- gratuitous inducers*
- isopropylthiogalactoside (IPTG)*
- constitutive mutation*

- repressor gene*
- operator region*
- operon model*
- repressor molecule*
- allosteric*
- negative control*
- merozygote
- $I^+, I^-, I^S, I^q, O^+, O^C$
- isolation of the repressor*
- equilibrium dialysis

- **Positive Control of the *lac* Operon***
  - catabolite-activating protein (CAP)*
  - catabolite repression
  - cyclic adenosine monophosphate (cAMP)*
  - adenyl cyclase*
  - cAMP-CAP complex*

- **Tryptophan (*trp*) Operon ***
  - tryptophan synthase*
  - normally inactive repressor
  - corepressor*
  - repressor-tryptophan complex*
  - repressor gene (*trpR*)
  - leader sequence*

- **RNA Regulates Gene Expression***
  - attenuation*
  - hairpin

- antiterminator hairpin*
- terminator hairpin*
- attenuator*
- UGG triplets*
- riboswitches*
- 5′-untranslated regions (UTRs)*
- terminator structure
- aptamer
- expression platform
- default conformation*
- antiterminator conformation*
- terminator conformation*
- small, noncoding RNAs (sRNAs)*
- positive and negative regulators

- **Adaptive Bacterial Immune System**
  - innate immunity*
  - adaptive immunity*
  - CRISPR
  - spacer*
  - CRISPR-associated (*cas*) genes
  - CRISPR-Cas*
  - spacer acquisition*
  - leader sequence*
  - CRISPR-derived RNAs (crRNAs)
  - crRNA biogenesis*
  - target interference*
  - Cas9

F15.1 Illustration of general processes of *negative* and *positive* control. If *negative* control is operating, the regulatory protein inhibits transcription. With *positive* control, transcription is stimulated.

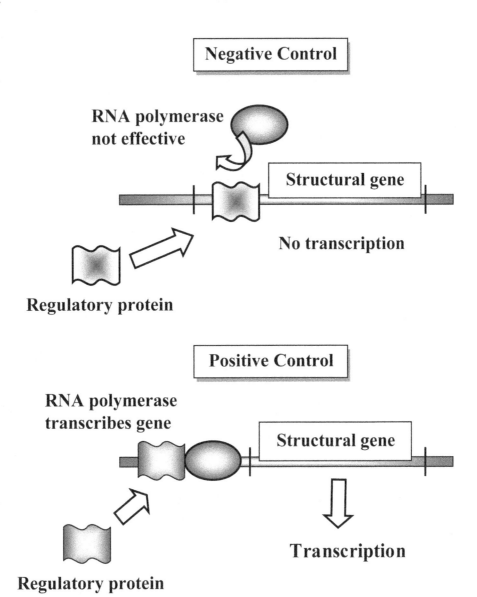

F15.2 Illustration of the nature of the product of the *I* gene. It can act "at a distance" because it is a protein that can diffuse through the cytoplasm and thus act in *trans*. There is no protein product of the operator sequence; therefore, it can act only in *cis*.

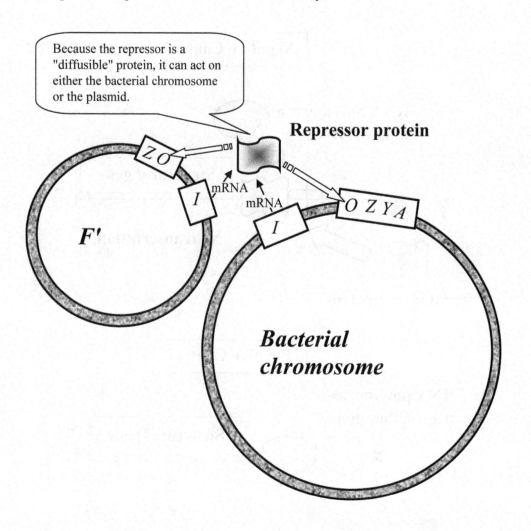

F15.3 Model of regulatory system described in problem 14. This is an example of *positive* control.

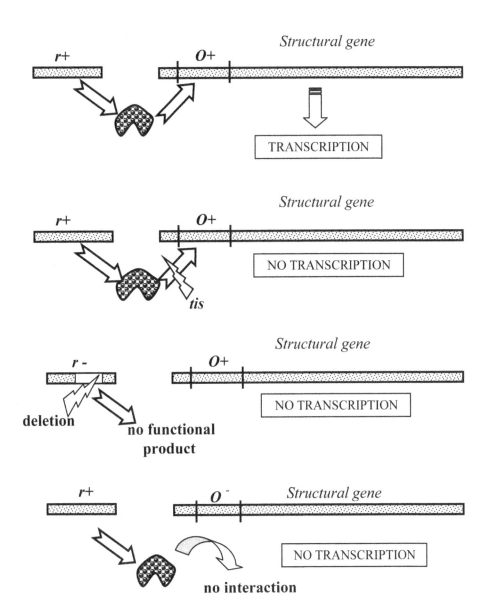

Answers to Now Solve This

15.1 (a) A one-nucleotide deletion early in the *lac Z* gene will cause a shift of the reading frame established by the *lac Z* initiator codon, resulting in a gene product whose sequence will be extremely altered or truncated. A cell with this mutation will not grow on a lactose medium because it cannot produce functional *β*-galactosidase. The reading frames for the *lac Y* gene and the *lac A* gene will be unaffected because each has its own initiator codon.

(b) The *A* gene product will likely be impaired, but this will not influence the cell's use of lactose as a carbon source.

15.2 To understand this question, it is necessary that you understand the negative regulation of the *lactose* operon by the *lac* repressor, as well as the positive control exerted by the CAP protein. Remember that lactose, when present, inactivates the *lac* repressor. Furthermore, glucose, when present, inhibits adenyl cyclase, which lowers cAMP levels and thereby reduces the positive action of CAP on the *lac* operon.

(a) With no lactose and no glucose, the operon is off because the *lac* repressor is bound to the operator. Although CAP is bound to its binding site, it will not override the action of the repressor.

(b) With lactose added to the medium, the *lac* repressor is inactivated, and the operon is transcribing the structural genes. With no glucose, CAP is bound to its binding site, thus enhancing transcription.

(c) With no lactose present in the medium, the *lac* repressor is bound to the operator region, and because glucose inhibits adenyl cyclase, CAP will not interact with its binding site. The operon is therefore "off."

(d) With lactose present, the *lac* repressor is inactivated; however, because glucose is also present, CAP will not interact with its binding site. Under this condition, transcription is severely diminished.

Chapter 15 Regulation of Gene Expression in Bacteria

Solutions to Problems and Discussion Questions

1. (a) From 1900 on, scientists have known that when certain additives are supplied to growth media, organisms respond with the production of certain enzymes. Such enzymes were referred to as inducible in contrast to constitutive enzymes that are made regardless of particular medium additives.

(b) Beginning with studies by Monod in 1946, it was determined that when lactose is added to a medium, *E. coli* respond with the production of enzymes involved in lactose metabolism. When lactose is removed, such enzymes decrease in concentration.

(c) Scientists identified constitutive mutants that produced lactose-metabolizing enzymes even in the absence of lactose. The first such mutant gene mapped close to the *lac* structural genes. Since the operon was active in the absence of the gene product and repressed when the gene was wild type, it was concluded that the gene encoded a repressor.

(d) Radioactive IPTG, a sulfur-containing analog of lactose, was shown to bind to the *lac* repressor. Extracts of I^- constitutive cells, having no *lac* repressor activity, did not bind IPTG. The IPTG-binding substance was shown to be a protein using labeled (radioactive sulfur) amino acids.

(e) For the *lac* system, addition of lactose to the medium causes the synthesis of *lac*-utilizing structural proteins. In contrast, when tryptophan is added to the medium, no tryptophan biosynthetic enzymes are produced.

2. Your essay should include a description of the evolutionary advantages of the efficient response to environmental resources and challenges (antibiotics, for example) when such compounds are present. Also discuss the advantages of the ability to turn off metabolic functions when they are not needed. Finally, include the advantages of having related functions in operons.

3. Under *negative* control, the regulatory molecule interferes with transcription, whereas in *positive* control, the regulatory molecule stimulates transcription. Furthermore, negative control requires that a molecule be removed from the DNA for transcription to occur, whereas positive control requires that a molecule be provided to the DNA for transcription to occur. Refer to F15.1 in this handbook for illustrations of both types of control. Examples of negative control are seen in the *lactose* and *tryptophan* systems while the action of the catabolite-activating protein (CAP) is an example of positive regulation.

4. In an *inducible system*, the repressor that normally interacts with the operator to inhibit transcription is inactivated by an *inducer*, thus permitting transcription. In a *repressible system*, a normally inactive repressor is *activated* by a corepressor. The activated repressor will bind to the operator to inhibit transcription. Because the interaction between the protein (repressor) and the DNA has a negative influence on transcription, the systems described here are forms of *negative control* (see F15.1 in this handbook).

5. Refer to the text and to F15.1 and F15.2 in this handbook to get a good understanding of the lactose system before starting.

$I^+O^+Z^+$ = **Inducible** because a repressor protein can interact with the operator to turn off transcription.

$I^-O^+Z^+$ = **Constitutive** because the repressor gene is mutant; therefore, no repressor protein is available.

$I^-O^CZ^+$ = **Constitutive** for two reasons. First, because the repressor gene is mutant, no repressor protein is available. Second, the operator sequence is mutant and could not bind repressor proteins even if any were present.

$I^-O^CZ^+/F'O^+$ = **Constitutive** because there is no functional repressor and there is a constitutive operator next to a normal Z gene (see F15.2 in this handbook).

$I^+O^CZ^+/F'O^+$ = **Constitutive** because there is a constitutive operator (O^C) next to a normal Z gene on the bacterial chromosome. This operator functions in *cis* and is not influenced by the repressor protein, thus constitutive synthesis of β-galactosidase will occur.

$I^SO^+Z^+$ = **Repressed** because the product of the I^S gene is *insensitive* to the inducer lactose and thus cannot be inactivated. The repressor will continually interact with the operator and will shut off transcription regardless of the presence or absence of lactose.

$I^SO^+Z^+/F'I^+$ = **Repressed.** As in the previous case, the product of the I^S gene is insensitive to the inducer lactose and thus cannot be inactivated. The repressor will continually interact with the operator and shut off transcription regardless of the presence or absence of lactose. The fact that there is a normal I^+ gene is of no consequence because once a repressor from I^S binds to an operator, the presence of normal repressor molecules will make no difference.

6. Refer to the text and to F15.2 in this handbook for a good understanding of the lactose system before starting.

$I^+ O^+ Z^+$ = Because there is an active repressor from the I^+ gene and no lactose to influence its function, there will be **no enzyme made**.

$I^+ O^C Z^+$ = There will be a **functional enzyme made** because the constitutive operator is in *cis* with a functional Z gene. The lactose in the medium will have no influence because the repressor cannot bind to the constitutive operator.

$I^- O^+ Z^-$ = There will be a **nonfunctional enzyme made**. The presence of the I^- gene makes the system constitutive, but the Z gene is mutant. The absence of lactose in the medium will have no influence because the nonfunctional repressor cannot bind to the operator.

$I^- O^+ Z^-$ = There will be a **nonfunctional enzyme made**: the system is constitutive (because of the I^- gene), but the Z gene is mutant. The lactose in the medium will have no influence because of the nonfunctional repressor, which cannot bind to the operator.

$I^- O^+ Z^+/F' I^+$ = There will be **no enzyme made**. In the absence of lactose, the functional repressor protein (the product of the I^+ gene provided by the F-factor) will bind to the operator and inhibit transcription.

$I^+ O^C Z^+/F' O^+$ = Because there is a constitutive operator in *cis* with a normal Z gene, there will be a **functional enzyme made**. The lactose in the medium will have no influence because of the mutant operator.

$I^+ O^+ Z^-/F' I^+ O^+ Z^+$ = There is lactose in the medium, so the repressor protein will not bind to the operator and transcription will occur. The presence of both a normal Z gene (provided by the F-factor) and mutant chromosomal Z gene allows both a **functional and a nonfunctional enzyme to be made**. The repressor protein is diffusible, working in *trans*.

$I^- O^+ Z^-/F' I^+ O^+ Z^+$ = There is no lactose in the medium, therefore the repressor protein (from the I^+ gene provided by the F-factor) will repress both operators and there will be **no enzyme made**.

$I^S O^+ Z^+/F' O^+$ = The product of the I^S gene is a superrepressor, which will bind to the operator. **No enzyme will be made**. The lack of lactose in the medium is of no consequence because the mutant repressor is insensitive to lactose.

$I^+ O^C Z^+/F' O^+ Z^+$ = The arrangement of the constitutive operator (O^C) with the wild-type Z gene will cause a **functional enzyme to be made**. Notice that the presence of lactose in the medium will allow for synthesis of functional enzyme from the plasmid as well.

7. The mutations described are consistent with the structure of the *lac* repressor. The 5′ upstream region contains the promoter, which needs to be intact for the gene to be transcribed. A nonfunctional promoter is consistent with the lack of a protein product in *lac I⁻* mutants. The more downstream sequences code for the protein, including the DNA-binding domain. A mutation here could give a superrepressor, such as that seen in *lac I^S* mutants.

8. While a single wild-type *E. coli* cell contains very few molecules of the *lac* repressor, cells with the *lac I^q* mutation make 10 times more repressor. This greater yield facilitated its isolation. Repressor binds to the gratuitous inducer, IPTG. Gilbert and Müller-Hill took advantage of this property and used equilibrium dialysis of extracts from *lac I^q* cells against radioactive IPTG. The material that bound the IPTG was identified as the repressor. Extracts of *lac I⁻* cells did not contain a component that bound to the labeled IPTG.

9. Since the repressor is encoded by DNA and is diffusible (it works *in trans*), it could be either RNA or protein. At that time, gene products were assumed to be proteins, and the *trans* aspect strengthened the thought that a protein was involved. Once the repressor was identified and purified, it was shown to have characteristics of protein, including the ability to be labeled by radioactive sulfur.

Evidence that the isolated protein serves as the *lac* repressor includes the following: First, a component in extracts from *lac I^q* cells could bind to labeled IPTG, whereas this component was missing in extracts from *lac I⁻* cells. Second, radioactive IPTG-binding protein was found to bind to DNA from λ phage that contained the *lac O⁺* region and not to other DNA sequences, indicating that the binding was specific. Third, additional experiments showed that the protein did not bind to DNA with the O^C mutation.

10. (a) Activated CAP exerts positive control over the *lac* operon. When present, CAP facilitates the binding of RNA polymerase to the *lac* promoter, thereby increasing the efficiency of transcription. The absence of a functional *crp* gene would, therefore, compromise the positive control exhibited by CAP and transcription of the operon would never be maximal.

(b) Without a CAP-binding site, the outcome would be similar to that described in part (a): there would be a reduction in the inducibility of the *lac* operon.

11. Because the four genes for erythritol catabolism are closely spaced and appear to be under coordinate control, an operon is likely to be involved. The product of the *eryD* gene is probably involved in repressing a promoter site. The system is induced when erythritol interrupts the action of the *eryD* repressor. These data are consistent with an inducible system of regulation.

12. Attenuation functions to reduce the synthesis of tryptophan when it is in full supply by reducing transcription of the *tryptophan* operon. The same effect is observed when tryptophan activates the repressor to shut off transcription of the *tryptophan* operon.

13. For both attenuation and riboswitches, regulation is mediated by RNA secondary structure, whereas regulation of the *lac* operon is mediated by a repressor protein.

14. Refer to F15.3 in this handbook for illustrations of the regulatory system described by this question. Because the deletion of the regulatory gene, *R*, causes a loss of synthesis of the enzymes, the regulatory gene product can be viewed as one that exerts *positive control*.

(a) In wild-type cells, when the regulatory molecule, tisophane (tis), is absent (F15.3, first panel), the regulatory protein (R) is free to bind to the operator where it promotes transcription. When tis is present (F15.3, second panel), no enzymes are made; therefore, tis must inactivate R. This could be accomplished if the binding of tis induces a conformational change in R that prevents its binding to the operator region.

(b) Mutations in the *R* gene prevent functional R proteins from being made. Since R is a positive regulator, its absence will prevent transcription (F15.3, third panel). Similarly, mutations in the operator would prevent binding of R, even in the absence of tis, thereby preventing transcription (F15.3, fourth panel).

15. Small noncoding RNAs (sRNAs) act by binding to mRNAs, usually at the 5′-end. If the sRNA binds to the ribosome-binding site (RBS), translation will be blocked. In some transcripts, however, the RBS is masked by the formation of internal secondary structure in the mRNA. In these cases, binding of sRNAs to a site adjacent to the RBS prevents formation of the mRNA secondary structure and unmasks the RBS, allowing translation.

16. Innate immunity describes cellular defense mechanisms that are not targeted to a specific pathogen. By contrast, adaptive immunity describes an evolving mechanism whereby exposure to a pathogen results in improved defense upon subsequent exposure to that same pathogen. The CRISPR-Cas system, which allows bacteria to become resistant to a given phage, exemplifies adaptive immunity.

17. A bacterial cell acquires spacer sequences that are derived from the genome of an invading virus and "stores" them in the CRISPR locus. Upon reinfection by that virus, the CRISPR locus is transcribed and processed into smaller CRISPR-derived RNAs (crRNAs), one of which contains the sequence derived from the invading virus. This mature crRNA complexes with a Cas nuclease and directs it to the complementary sequence in the viral genome, where the nuclease cleaves viral DNA.

18. With each infection by a different type of phage, the bacterial cell acquires viral sequences, which are added as spacers to the bacterial CRISPR locus. Each sequence is added proximal to the leader sequence, so newer sequences are closer to the leader and older sequences are more distant. Such stored "trophies," therefore, provide scientists not only with the identities of phages that the bacterial cell encountered previously but also the order in which they were encountered. Because these spacers are mobilized to direct a protective response by the bacterial cell, scientists can use them to predict the cell's phage immunities and sensitivities.

Chapter 16: Regulation of Gene Expression in Eukaryotes

Concept Areas	Corresponding Problems
Overview of Eukaryotic Gene Regulation	1, 2, 3, 4
DNA Methylation	1
Nuclear Organization	4
Chromatin Structure and Proteins	5, 6, 8, 27
Transcription Factors	1, 8, 28
Promoters, Enhancers, and Silencers	1, 7, 8, 9, 10, 11, 27
Splicing	1, 12, 13, 14
mRNA Stability	15, 16
RNAi	1, 17, 18, 19, 20, 21, 22
Translational and Posttranslational Regulation	23, 24, 25
RNA/Protein Localization	23, 24
Protein Degradation	26, 29

Structures and Processes Checklist—Significant items that deserve special attention are identified with a "*".

(Check topic when mastered–provide examples where appropriate–understand the context of each entry)

- ○ **Overview**
  - ○ cell-specific expression
  - ○ temporal-specific expression
  - ○ consequences of misregulation
- ○ **Organization of the Eukaryotic Cell**
  - ○ positive and negative regulation
  - ○ multiple levels of regulation*
  - ○ DNA associated with proteins*
  - ○ spatial separation of processes*
  - ○ mRNAs processed*
  - ○ modulation of translation
  - ○ posttranslational modifications
- ○ **Chromatin Modifications***
  - ○ histones and nonhistone proteins

- ○ chromatin*
- ○ nucleosomes
- ○ 30-nm fibers
- ○ chromosome territory*
- ○ interchromatin compartments*
- ○ nuclear architecture
- ○ inhibitory, or closed, conformation*
- ○ open chromatin*
- ○ histone variants*
- ○ H2A vs. H2A.Z
- ○ histone modifications*
- ○ histone acetyltransferase (HAT) enzymes*
- ○ activator proteins

154

- ○ histone deacetylase (HDACs)*
- ○ repressor proteins
- ○ chromatin remodeling complexes*
- ○ repositioned nucleosomes
- ○ DNA methylation*
- ○ 5-methylcytosine
- ○ CG doublet
- ○ CpG island*
- ○ represses gene expression
- ○ **Eukaryotic Transcription**
  - ○ three RNA polymerases
  - ○ *cis*-acting elements*
  - ○ *trans*-acting factors*
  - ○ promoter*
  - ○ transcription start site
  - ○ core promoter
  - ○ proximal promoter elements*
  - ○ focused core promoters*
  - ○ dispersed core promoters*
  - ○ housekeeping genes
  - ○ core-promoter elements*
  - ○ Initiator element (Inr)*
  - ○ TATA box*
  - ○ TFIIB recognition element (BRE)*
  - ○ motif ten element (MTE)
  - ○ downstream promoter element (DPE)
  - ○ CAAT box*
- ○ GC box
- ○ enhancer*
- ○ tissue- or temporal-specificity
- ○ position independent
- ○ variable orientation
- ○ silencer*
- ○ **Eukaryotic Transcription Initiation**
  - ○ transcription factors
  - ○ general transcription factors (GTF)*
  - ○ activators*
  - ○ repressors*
  - ○ fine-tuning
  - ○ human metallothionein 2A (*MT2A*) gene*
- ○ **Activators, Repressors, and Chromatin Structure**
  - ○ RNAP II*
  - ○ pre-initiation complex (PIC)*
  - ○ TFIIA, TFIIB, TFIID, TFIIE, TFIIF, TFIIH
  - ○ Mediator
  - ○ TBP (TATA Binding Protein)
  - ○ TAFs (TBP Associated Factors)
  - ○ DNA loops*
  - ○ recruitment model
  - ○ coactivators
  - ○ enhanceosome*
  - ○ chromatin alterations model
  - ○ nuclear relocation model

Chapter 16: Regulation of Gene Expression in Eukaryotes

- **Regulation of Alternative Splicing**
  - spliceform
  - alternative splicing*
  - isoform*
  - *Mhc* gene
  - types of alternative splicing*
  - cassette exons
  - alternative splice site
  - intron retention
  - mutually exclusive exons
  - alternative promoters
  - alternative polyadenylation
  - calcitonin/calcitonin gene-related peptide (*CT/CGRP*) gene*
  - proteome*
  - *Dscam* gene
  - 38,016 different proteins possible
  - splicing enhancers
  - RNA-binding proteins (RBPs)*
  - tissue-specific expression
  - spliceopathies*
  - myotonic dystrophy (DM)*
  - DM1, DM2
  - expansion of repeat sequences
  - sequester splicing regulators
- **mRNA Stability***
  - steady-state level
  - exoribonucleases
- deadenylation-dependent decay*
- deadenylases
- exosome complex
- decapping enzymes*
- XRN1*
- deadenylation-independent decay*
- endoribonucleases*
- premature stop codon
- mRNA surveillance*
- nonsense-mediated decay (NMD)*
- **Posttranscriptional Regulation**
  - noncoding RNAs (ncRNAs)*
  - RNA interference (RNAi)*
  - small noncoding RNAs (sncRNAs)*
  - small interfering RNAs (siRNAs)*
  - microRNA (miRNA)*
  - Dicer*
  - RNA-induced silencing complex (RISC)*
  - Argonaute
  - primary miRNAs (pri-miRNAs)*
  - hairpin structure
  - Drosha
  - pre-miRNAs*
  - miRNA response elements (MREs)
  - knockdown of gene function*
  - Patisiran
  - long noncoding RNAs (lncRNAs)*

- competing endogenous RNAs (ceRNAs)*
- bind miRNAs

○ **mRNA Localization**

- asymmetric protein distribution*
- zip code*
- zip code binding protein 1 (ZBP1)*
- Src
- ZBP1 phosphorylation*

○ **Regulation of Protein Activity**

- posttranslational modification*
- covalent modification
- kinases
- phosphatases
- target for degradation*
- ubiquitin
- ubiquitination*
- proteasome*
- ubiquitin ligases

Chapter 16: Regulation of Gene Expression in Eukaryotes

Answers to Now Solve This

16.1 Tumor suppressors, such as *BRCA1*, normally act to regulate cell-cycle checkpoints or the initiation of apoptosis, both of which prevent accumulation of DNA damage in cells. Likewise, DNA repair proteins, such as *MLH1*, function to prevent gene mutations. If either of these genes were to be suppressed by methylation at their promoter, cells with damaged DNA will continue to proliferate, and the frequency of mutation would continue to increase because the DNA repair system is compromised. These resulting increases in mutations might occur in tumor-suppressor genes or proto-oncogenes, thereby promoting cancer.

16.2 General transcription factors associate with a promoter to stimulate transcription of a specific gene. Some *trans*-acting elements, when bound to enhancers (for example the ER protein), interact with coactivators (estrogen, in this example) to enhance transcription by forming an enhanceosome, which stimulates transcription initiation. Transcription can be repressed by a similar mechanism when proteins bind to silencer DNA elements and generate repressive chromatin structures. The same molecule may bind to a different chromosomal regulatory site (enhancer or silencer), depending on the molecular environment of a given tissue type.

16.3 RISC searches for target mRNAs, guided by single-stranded miRNA molecules. These guide RNAs recruit RISC to the proper targets by binding to complementary sequences (miRNA response elements, or MREs) in the mRNA. If the miRNA and message are perfectly matched, RISC cleaves the target mRNA in the middle of the double-stranded sequence, leading to message degradation. In the case where the miRNA is a partial match, translation is blocked.

16.4 Without the zip code sequence, the actin mRNA would not be bound by ZBP1 and, consequently, would neither be silenced nor transported. As a result, actin would be produced in the cytoplasm near the nucleus and not in the lamellipodium.

Chapter 16: Regulation of Gene Expression in Eukaryotes

Solutions to Problems and Discussion Questions

1. (a) Eukaryotic cells have a different cellular organization than do bacteria. In eukaryotes, genomic DNA resides in the nucleus, whereas ribosomes, the translational machinery, reside in the cytoplasm. RNA is synthesized in the nucleus, exported to the cytoplasm, then translated by ribosomes. This means that transcription and translation are separated both spatially and temporally.

(b) First, for a particular region of a chromosome, there is an inverse relationship between the degree of DNA methylation and the degree of gene expression. Second, large chromosomal regions that are silent (such as the X chromosome) are heavily methylated. In addition, if methylation is blocked, those genes become activated.

(c) Core promoter elements are the staging area for the assembly of the pre-initiation complex. Mutations within promoters alter transcription efficiencies. (See Figure 16.4 in the textbook.)

(d) Experiments have shown that promoters must be in a specific orientation, immediately upstream of the gene for transcription to occur. By contrast, similar experiments that reversed the orientation of enhancer elements showed that such a change had no effect on enhancer function.

(e) Scientists compared the activities of protein isoforms from different tissues by experimentally replacing one isoform by another. For example, Bernstein and Maughan studied the embryonic and flight muscle isoforms of the contractile protein produced by alternatively spliced transcripts of the *Mhc* gene in *Drosophila.* The embryonic form, when expressed in flight muscles, caused the flies to beat their wings at a lower frequency.

(f) In both animals and plants, scientists showed that complementary base pairing between miRNA and its target mRNA led to downregulation of the protein encoded by that mRNA for such diverse processes as cell-cycle regulation, development, and nerve function.

2. Your essay should include a description of the identity and nature of each type of *cis* element, the action of the *trans*-acting protein(s), and the consequence of this action.

3. Eukaryotic DNA is associated with various proteins, including histones and nonhistone chromosomal proteins. The positioning and strength of binding of nucleosomes offer a means of regulating DNA accessibility to RNA polymerase that is not available in bacteria. In addition, bacterial transcription and translation are coupled because the processes are not spatially separated. By contrast, eukaryotic chromosomes reside in the nucleus, and the nuclear membrane separates, both temporally and spatially, the processes of transcription and translation. This provides an opportunity for posttranscriptional, pre-translational regulation. Furthermore, while bacteria respond genetically to changes in their external environment, cells of multicellular eukaryotes interact with each other as well as with the external environment. The structural and functional diversities of cell types of a multicellular eukaryote, coupled with the finding that all cells of an organism contain a complete complement of genes, suggest that in some cells certain genes are active that are not active in other cells.

4. Chromosomes occupy discrete domains called chromosome territories, which are separated by channels, called interchromatin compartments. Active genes are found at territory edges, and transcripts are moved into the interchromatin compartments for processing. Nuclear pores adjoin to these compartments, which facilitates transport of mRNA from the nucleus.

5. A major modification of histones involves acetylation by histone acetyltransferases and deacetylation by histone deacetylases. Acetylation creates more "open" chromatin, which allows transcription, whereas deacetylation restores chromatin to a more "closed" state.

6. One form of remodeling is the use of histone variants, such as H2A.Z, which makes DNA-nucleosome interactions less stable and chromatin more open. In addition, large remodeling complexes can be recruited to promoters to reposition nucleosomes along the DNA. Alterations that create a more open chromatin conformation will allow transcription, whereas downregulation of transcription will result if a more closed conformation is created.

7. *Promoters* are conserved DNA sequences that influence transcription from the "upstream" (5′) side of mRNA coding genes. Promoters are bound by transcription factors and RNAP II. Core promoters contain the start site and the minimal sequence motifs

(Inr, TATA box, BRE, MTE, and DPE) needed for accurate transcription initiation. Proximal promoter elements (CAAT box and GC box) are located farther upstream and contain binding sites that influence transcription efficiency. *Enhancers* are *cis*-acting sequences that increase the rate of transcription of a gene and may confer temporal and tissue specificity. Unlike promoters, the position of the enhancer need not be fixed; it may be significantly upstream, downstream, or within the gene being regulated. Further, enhancer orientation may be inverted without significantly influencing its action.

8. In general, activators and repressors change the relationship of RNAP II to the transcription complex. DNA loops are thought to bring distant enhancer or silencer elements into proximity with promoter regions of the genes under their regulation. Activators can increase either the rate of preinitiation complex assembly or its stability, or they can increase the rate of release of RNAP II from the promoter. Repressors function conversely or block the promoter. Both factors can also alter chromatin structure. Activators can recruit histone acetyltransferases or chromatin remodeling complexes to DNA loops to make the DNA more accessible, whereas repressors can recruit histone deacetylases or chromatin remodelers to close the chromatin conformation.

9. Generally, one determines the influence of various regulatory elements by removing necessary elements or adding extra elements. In addition, examining the outcome of mutations within such elements often provides insight as to function. Assay systems determine the relative levels of gene expression after such alterations.

10. *Focused* promoters specify a single transcription initiation site, whereas for *dispersed* promoters, there are many weak initiation sites that cover a relatively large region (50 to 100 nucleotides). Most genes of lower eukaryotes use focused transcription and in general are genes that are highly regulated. Dispersed promoters are more often associated with genes that act constitutively. They direct expression from approximately 70 percent of vertebrate genes.

11. Inr, BRE, DPE, and MTE sequences are double-stranded core-promoter elements that are needed for accurate initiation. The Initiator element (Inr) is a pyrimidine-rich approximately six-nucleotide sequence that includes the transcription start site. BRE (or the TFIIB recognition element) is immediately upstream or downstream from the TATA box while

MTE (the motif ten element) and DPE (the downstream promoter element) are downstream from the transcription site (+18 to +27 and +28 to +33, respectively). While Inr and BRE are present in all focused promoters, MTF and DPE are present only in some.

12. Your text describes six different patterns used, as described below.

cassette exons—Whole exons are excluded from the mature message, resulting in a protein that is missing certain sequences (perhaps an entire protein domain).

alternative splice sites within an exon—Certain sequences are either included or excluded. This can generate proteins with different sequences or may be important for gene regulatory events.

intron retention—Introns are included in the mature mRNAs. They can be translated to produce novel isoforms or used to promote mRNA degradation or sequestration.

mutually exclusive exons—Different versions of an exon exist that allow for the presence of different domains in the protein.

alternative promoters—Messages with different 5′ exons and proteins with different N-terminal ends are made.

alternative polyadenylation—Messages with different 3′ coding sequences as well as different 3′ untranslated regions, which can be important in regulatory events, are made.

13. The use of a cassette exon and alternative polyadenylation results in production of two mRNAs from the CT/CGRP pre-mRNA. In the message encoding the CT protein, exon 4, which contains a polyadenylation signal, is present. The resulting protein contains only the first four exons. In the second mRNA, the message encoding the CGRP protein, exon 4 is skipped, and the polyadenylation signal from a downstream exon is used. The resulting protein contains exons 1-3 plus exons 5 and 6.

14. Promoters mark transcriptional start sites, which, by definition, exist at the 5′ end of the transcript. A gene with multiple alternative promoters would, therefore, produce transcripts with different 5′ ends. Depending on which promoter-containing exon is used and its location relative to other exons in the gene, other sequence differences could also exist.

Similarly, polyadenylation signals mark transcriptional stop sites at the 3′ ends of genes. Once such a signal is encountered, transcription is terminated and downstream exons are not included in the message. When alternative polyadenylation signals are used, the exon containing the first signal is skipped, allowing previously excluded exons to be transcribed and resulting in a message with a different 3′-end.

15. The 7mG-cap at the 5′-end and the 3′-poly-A tail present on eukaryotic messages serve to protect these RNAs from the actions of exoribonucleases. These structures must be removed to initiate mRNA decay. Deadenylases, which function in deadenylation-dependent decay, shorten the poly-A tail and lead to the recruitment of either a degradative exosome complex or decapping enzymes. Decapping enzymes function in both deadenylation-dependent and -independent decay, by removing the 5′-cap and allowing XRN1 exonuclease degradation.

16. Normally, stop codons are located near the poly-A tail of the message or downstream of exon-exon junctions. Termination signals that do not meet these criteria are considered by the cell as premature.

17. The action of RNAi depends on complementary base-pairing; therefore, gene silencing occurs in a sequence-specific manner. Furthermore, RNAi is considered potent because only a few molecules are needed to degrade large amounts of target mRNA or to prevent its translation.

18. In general terms, a cytoplasmic protein, Dicer, processes double-stranded small noncoding RNA (sncRNA) molecules to produce shorter dsRNAs. These associate with RISC (RNA-induced silencing complex), where an Argonaut-family protein cleaves and discards one of the two strands. The retained strand guides RISC to the complementary target message, where the complex acts to prevent expression. The specific mechanism of silencing depends on the type of sncRNA used.

19. Similarities: Both types of RNAi begin with double-stranded sncRNAs that are processed to a smaller size by Dicer. These smaller RNAs associate with RISC, which retains only one strand. This strand is used by RISC as a guide to the target mRNA sequence. Finally, cleavage of the resulting double-stranded RNAi/mRNA can occur and lead to message degradation.

Differences: (1) *Source of the dsRNA*—For siRNA, the longer dsRNA originates from viral infection or from transposons. miRNAs, however, are encoded by the cell and transcribed in the nucleus. (2) *Processing of the longer RNAs*—Primary miRNAs undergo processing (capping, polyadenylation, and sometimes splicing) whereas siRNAs do not. (3) *Secondary structure*—Pri-miRNAs form hairpins that are processed by Drosha prior to their exportation from the nucleus. The dsRNA for siRNA does not form this secondary structure as part of its mechanism. (4) *Mechanism of silencing*—The only outcome for RNAi mediated by siRNA is message degradation, while there are two outcomes, message degradation or blocking of translation, for miRNA-mediated RNAi.

20. Because miRNA must hybridize by base pairing with its target to direct RISC to the correct message, you can determine the sequence that is complementary to the miRNA and search for that sequence among the cellular mRNAs, whose sequences are also known.

21. A number of viruses use RNA as their genome rather than DNA. If the genome consists of dsRNA, siRNA molecules could be generated directly from this genomic RNA using the cellular enzyme, Dicer. If the genome consists of ssRNA, virally encoded replicase could synthesize a complementary RNA strand, producing a dsRNA molecule. Dicer could then generate siRNA molecules, as above.

22. ceRNAs are long noncoding RNAs that contain miRNA response elements (MREs). MREs are sequences that are complementary to miRNA and that serve as miRNA binding sites. When present, ceRNAs will compete with mRNA targets for binding of miRNA molecules, rendering the miRNA less effective.

23. Certain protein functions may be needed in only a specific subcellular location rather than throughout the cytoplasm-either to serve a specific mechanical or structural function or for the establishment of protein gradients. Messages for these specialized proteins are transported in a translationally inert state to the proper location, then released and activated for translation. This requires the coordinated interplay among *cis*-acting elements and RBPs in the nucleus, the cytoskeleton and its motor proteins in the cytoplasm, and a protein-modification protein at the destination. The example given in your text describes the transport of actin mRNA to the lamellipodia of neurons. Look over this example and identify the specific components that fulfill the requirements described above.

24. Even though a particular species of mRNA might be distributed in a fairly uniform fashion throughout a cell, it does not follow that it is uniformly translated. It is likely that the mRNA is bound by an RBP that prevents translation. A modification of the RBP that changes its conformation (phosphorylation, for example) would be needed to remove the RBP and allow translation. The modifying enzyme would need to be localized to specific subcellular locations to result in disperse mRNA distribution but localized protein production.

25. Phosphorylation of a protein usually brings about a conformational change that alters the function or activity of that protein. There is no general "rule" describing the absolute effect of phosphorylation on function. For example, phosphorylation will activate some enzymes and inactivate others; it will induce binding by some proteins and prevent binding by others. The results of phosphorylation are easily reversed by the removal of the phosphate group by phosphatases.

26. The proteasome degrades only proteins that carry a poly-ubiquitin tag. Because this tag is added by ubiquitin ligase, it could be said that the proteasome is indirectly regulated by ubiquitin ligase.

27. Upon experiencing hypoxia, DNA looping brings the promoter and enhancer into proximity. This allows an activator protein (HIF) to recruit a coactivator (p300) to an enhancer of the EPO-encoding gene and, thereby, near to the promoter. Being a histone acetyl transferase, p300 can catalyze the acetylation of histones at the promoter of the EPO-encoding gene, which "opens' the chromatin conformation and promotes transcription.

28. (a) As a transcription factor, TBX20 helps to either upregulate or downregulate expression of genes involved in heart development, leading to a characteristic expression profile in wild-type cells. When the *Tbx20* gene is deleted, expression of those genes normally regulated by TBX20 will change. Thus, genes that are normally suppressed will be active and genes that are normally activated will be suppressed. Comparison of the transcriptomes of the two cell types will reflect these changes. A transcript that is normally activated by the transcription factor will be more prevalent in wild-type cells than in *Tbx20*

cells. Likewise, a transcript that is normally suppressed will be less prevalent in wild-type than in mutant cells.

(b) Opposite responses by different genes to the same transcription factor could be driven by the presence of different cofactors, different timing of activation vs. repression, or even the presence of different isoforms of TBX20.

29. (a) Given that ICP0 functions as a ubiquitin ligase, it is likely that ZEB1 and ZEB2 are poly-ubiquitinated and subsequently degraded by the proteasome.

(b) ZEB1 and ZEB2 are repressors. If they normally act to suppress expression from the miR-183 cluster, their elimination would result in the upregulation of the cluster.

(c) The miRNAs encoded by the miR-183 cluster could serve to downregulate expression of genes that protect against viral infection. If so, their activation by ICP0 would lead to an inability of the cell to mount a defense against HSV-1 infection and, therefore, allow the virus to proliferate.

Chapter 17: Recombinant DNA Technology

Concept Areas	Corresponding Problems
Making DNA Clones and Libraries	1, 2, 3, 4, 8, 9, 12
Restriction Endonucleases	2, 3, 6, 7, 9
Detecting Cloned Sequences	1, 10, 16, 20
Methods of Analysis of Cloned Sequences	16, 18, 19
DNA Sequencing	1, 15
Polymerase Chain Reaction	1, 11, 13, 14
Transgenic and Knockout Organisms	1, 17, 18, 19, 20, 21, 27
CRISPR-Cas	21, 22, 23, 24, 25, 26, 27
Applications	2, 4, 5, 8, 9, 12, 16, 22, 26

Structures and Processes Checklist–Significant items that deserve special attention are identified with a "*".

(Check topic when mastered–provide examples where appropriate–understand the context of each entry)

- ○ **Overview**
  - ○ recombinant DNA
  - ○ recombinant DNA technology
  - ○ clones
- ○ **Recombinant DNA Technology***
  - ○ restriction enzymes*
  - ○ cloning vector*
  - ○ recognition sequence*
  - ○ restriction site
  - ○ palindrome*
  - ○ cohesive ends*
  - ○ blunt-end fragments*
  - ○ *Escherichia coli**
  - ○ anneal*
  - ○ DNA ligase*
  - ○ cloning vectors
  - ○ key properties of vectors*
  - ○ restriction sites
- ○ independent replication
- ○ selectable marker gene
- ○ reporter gene
- ○ plasmid*
- ○ multiple cloning site
- ○ transformation*
- ○ electroporation*
- ○ origin of replication (*ori*)
- ○ *amp*^{R} gene*
- ○ *lacZ* gene*
- ○ blue-white screening*
- ○ ampicillin
- ○ X-gal*
- ○ insert limitations of plasmids
- ○ phage vectors
- ○ bacteriophage λ*
- ○ bacterial artificial chromosome (BAC)*

- ○ yeast artificial chromosome (YAC)*
- ○ expression vector
- ○ Ti plasmid*
- ○ **Collections of Cloned Sequences**
  - ○ DNA libraries
  - ○ genomic library*
  - ○ whole-genome sequencing*
  - ○ complementary DNA (cDNA) library*
  - ○ reverse transcription*
  - ○ oligo(dT) primer
  - ○ library screening*
  - ○ probe*
  - ○ hybridization*
  - ○ detection of probe*
  - ○ genomics
- ○ **Copying DNA**
  - ○ polymerase chain reaction (PCR)*
  - ○ primers*
  - ○ denaturation*
  - ○ 92-95°C
  - ○ hybridization/annealing of primers*
  - ○ 45-65°C
  - ○ extension*
  - ○ 65-75°C
  - ○ thermocycler
  - ○ thermostable DNA polymerase*
  - ○ *Taq* DNA polymerase*
  - ○ limitations of PCR*
  - ○ applications of PCR*
  - ○ reverse transcription PCR (RT-PCR)

- ○ quantitative real-time PCR (qPCR)
- ○ real-time PCR
- ○ **Molecular Techniques***
  - ○ agarose gel electrophoresis
  - ○ ethidium bromide
  - ○ restriction map
  - ○ hybridization*
  - ○ Southern blot analysis*
  - ○ Southern blotting
  - ○ Northern blot analysis *
  - ○ Northern blotting
  - ○ Western blotting*
  - ○ fluorescence *in situ* hybridization (FISH)*
  - ○ spectral karyotypes*
- ○ **DNA Sequencing***
  - ○ dideoxy chain-termination sequencing*
  - ○ Sanger sequencing
  - ○ deoxyribonucleotides (dNTPs)*
  - ○ dideoxynucleotides (ddNTPs)*
  - ○ read length
  - ○ sequence run
  - ○ capillary gel electrophoresis*
  - ○ computer-automated
  - ○ high-throughput DNA sequencing
  - ○ next-generation sequencing (NGS) technologies
  - ○ sequencing-by-synthesis (SBS)
  - ○ third-generation sequencing (TGS)
  - ○ single-molecule sequencing in real time (SMRT)
  - ○ RNA sequencing

- **Knockout and Transgenic Organisms**
  - gene targeting*
  - gene knockout (KO)*
  - loss-of-function mutation
  - double-knockout animals (DKOs)
  - triple-knockout animals (TKOs)
  - targeting vector
  - embryonic stem (ES) cells*
  - recombinase
  - pseudopregnant mouse
  - chimera
  - null mice
  - embryonic lethality
  - conditional knockout
  - transgenic animal
  - knock-in animal
  - humanized mice

- **CRISPR-Cas**
  - genome editing
  - CRISPR (clustered regularly interspaced palindromic repeats)-Cas
  - Cas9
  - protospacer-adjacent motif (PAM)
  - single guide RNA (sgRNA)
  - nonhomologous end-joining (NHEJ)
  - homology-directed repair (HDR)
  - indels
  - donor template
  - off-target edits
  - CRISPR-Cas applications

Answers to Now Solve This

17.1 (a) The transformation mixture will produce two types of transformed cells: those containing the recombinant plasmid and those containing recircularized plasmid (a cut plasmid whose ends religated without incorporation of an insert). In the recombinant plasmid, *Drosophila* DNA was cloned into the *Pst*I site, disrupting the ampicillin resistance gene of the plasmid, but leaving the tetracycline resistance gene intact. Therefore, any bacterium that contains the recombinant plasmid will be ampicillin-sensitive and tetracycline-resistant. In the nonrecombinant plasmid, both resistance genes are intact, and cells that take up this plasmid will be resistant to both antibiotics. Therefore, either antibiotic will select cells that have taken up a plasmid, but the population of cells selected by each will differ.

(b) Cells containing plasmids with the *Drosophila* insert will grow only on plates containing tetracycline. Cells that contain recircularized plasmid will be able to grow on any of the three media.

(c) Resistance to both antibiotics by a transformed bacterium could be explained in several ways. First, if digestion of the original plasmid by the *Pst*I enzyme was incomplete, then no change in biological properties of the uncut plasmids would be expected. Also, it is possible that the cut ends of the plasmid were ligated together in the original form with no insert.

17.2 Using the human nucleotide sequence, identify regions of the β-globin gene that are relatively conserved among mammals. Select sequences from these regions to create PCR primers and amplify the sequences from human DNA, thereby creating a probe to screen the okapi library. The probe will hybridize to complementary sequences in the library, thus identifying the library clone (or clones) that contains the sequence of interest. Alternatively, isolate DNA from the okapi library and use the primers to amplify the sequence directly. Next, sequence the amplified DNA, and compare the nucleotide and deduced amino sequences against their human counterparts.

Chapter 17 Recombinant DNA Technology

Solutions to Problems and Discussion Questions

1. (a) Plasmids that have incorporated DNA sequences will be larger than the original plasmid molecule. Therefore, the presumptive recombinant plasmid can be linearized (by digestion with a restriction enzyme that has a single recognition sequence in the plasmid) and its size determined by gel electrophoresis. In addition, one of the plasmid genes is generally inactivated, because the inserted DNA interrupts that gene. For example, if you insert a piece of DNA into the ampicillin resistance gene of a plasmid, the recombinant plasmid is no longer able to confer resistance to that antibiotic. Other techniques that involve "insertional mutagenesis" include blue-white screening. These techniques also serve to indicate whether host cells have been successfully transformed.

(b) Purified genomic DNA is first denatured and then specific primers are allowed to anneal. Once primers have annealed, they are extended by a DNA polymerase. Each resulting daughter molecule is used as a template for the next cycle of synthesis. The process is repeated to produce many copies of a specific DNA molecule.

(c) Next-generation sequencing utilizes simultaneous sequencing reactions in which thousands of identical template DNA fragments are immobilized on a solid surface and fluorescently labeled nucleotides are detected as they are incorporated. In third-generation sequencing methods, a single molecule of single-stranded DNA serves as a template. In one such strategy, the DNA polymerase is tethered in a nanopore and fluorescently labeled nucleotides are detected as they are incorporated. The overall goal is to increase the speed and accuracy of sequencing while reducing the per base cost.

(d) The three different techniques each change the genotype of an organism, some by disrupting or removing a functional gene (knockouts and editing), some by adding a new gene (transgenics and editing), and some by modifying an existing gene (editing). Analysis of the resulting phenotypic changes (if any) provides insight into gene functions.

2. Your essay should include an appreciation for the relative ease with which sections of DNA can be inserted into various vectors as well as for the amplification and isolation of such DNA. You should also include the possibilities of modifying recombinant molecules.

3. Recombinant DNA technology, also called gene splicing, involves the creation of DNA molecules that are not typically found in nature. *Restriction enzymes* cut DNA at specific sites and often yield single-stranded overhangs or "sticky" ends, which allow DNA molecules cut with the same enzyme to anneal to each other. A *vector* is a DNA molecule that is used to carry exogenous sequences of interest into host cells. Vectors may be plasmids, bacteriophage, or artificial chromosomes. Recombinant vectors can transform a *host cell* (bacterium, yeast cell, etc.) and be amplified in number. In a DNA cloning experiment, DNA ligase is used to "seal the nicks" (create covalent phosphodiester bonds) in the DNA backbone between inserted DNA and vector to yield an intact double-stranded DNA molecule. Restriction enzymes, by contrast, break phosphodiester bonds.

4. Even though the human gene coding for insulin contains introns, the processed mRNA does not. A cDNA that is free of introns can be generated from this mRNA by reverse transcription, cloned into plasmids, and used to transform bacteria. Because the transformed insulin genes are free of introns, no processing issues surface.

5. Although bacteria are commonly used in cloning, other cell types (such as yeast, insect, mammalian etc.) are also very useful. Bacteria do not process transcripts (or proteins) as eukaryotes do; therefore, there is often an advantage to using a eukaryotic host. In addition, one might be interested in the influence of a specific DNA segment in a specific host environment, thus necessitating the use of a variety of hosts.

6. This segment contains the palindromic sequence of GGATCC, which is recognized by the restriction enzyme *Bam*HI. It also contains the sequence of GATC, which is recognized by the restriction enzyme *Sau*3AI (see the "Insights and Solutions" box in the text). The double-stranded sequences are shown below:

GGATCC	GATC
CCTAGG	CTAG
*Bam*HI	*Sau*3AI

7. Classical restriction enzymes are dimers of identical units that, of course, recognize identical sequences. This allows a single enzyme to make simultaneous cuts on both strands of DNA.

8. Plasmids are small, so they are relatively easy to separate from the host bacterial chromosome. They have relatively few restriction sites and can be engineered fairly easily (i.e., polylinkers and reporter genes added). However, plasmids suffer from the limitation that they can only accept small DNA fragments and that they can use only bacteria as hosts. BACs are artificial bacterial chromosomes that can be engineered for certain qualities such as carrying large DNA fragments. YACs (yeast artificial chromosomes) are extensively used to clone DNA in yeast. They accept extremely large DNA inserts, ranging in size from 100 kb to 1000 kb. As a eukaryotic organism, yeast processes RNA and proteins, allowing the study of eukaryotic genes.

9. Using an enzyme with a relatively rare recognition site will produce larger fragments, which might be desired if one wanted to isolate intact genes or centromeres, and so on. The rarity of a sequence is sometimes related to its length. For example, assuming a random distribution of all four bases, a four-base sequence would occur (on average) every 256 base pairs (4^4), and a six-base sequence would occur every 4096 base pairs (4^6). This is akin to calculating the probability of any particular sequence of bases occurring in a row (of 4 or 6).

10. A probe is any DNA or RNA that is complementary to some part of a target gene or sequence. Probes are used to identify and/or locate a particular nucleic acid sequence among a pool of sequences.

11. The total number of molecules after 15 cycles would be 32,768, or $(2)^{15}$.

12. A cDNA library provides DNAs from mRNA transcripts and is useful in identifying what are likely to be functional DNAs. If one desires to examine noncoding as well as coding regions, a genomic library would be more useful.

13. (a) Heating to 92–95°C denatures the double-stranded DNA so that it dissociates into single strands. This usually takes about 1 minute.

(b) Lowering the temperature to 45–65°C allows the primers to bind to the denatured DNA.

(c) Bringing the temperature to 65–75°C allows the heat-stable DNA polymerase an opportunity to extend the primers by adding nucleotides to the 3′ ends of each growing strand. Each PCR reaction is designed with specific temperatures (not ranges) at each step, based on the characteristics of the DNAs (template and primers).

14. *Taq* polymerase is from a bacterium called *Thermus aquaticus*, which typically lives in hot springs. It is a heat-stable DNA polymerase that can tolerate extreme temperature changes.

15. Next-generation and third-generation sequencing methods can generate more sequence data in a shorter time frame, with a high degree of accuracy, and for a dramatically reduced cost. Third-generation methods offer the additional advantage of sequencing single DNA molecules, with a goal of even greater accuracy.

16. In FISH, a labeled probe is hybridized to a complementary stretch of DNA in a chromosome. As such, it can be used to locate a specific DNA sequence (often a gene or gene fragment) in a chromosome. Spectral karyotyping uses FISH to detect individual chromosomes, a distinct advantage in identifying chromosomal abnormalities.

17. A knockout animal has a piece of DNA missing, whereas a transgenic animal usually has a piece of DNA added.

18. If a transgene integrates into a coding or regulatory region of the genome, it is likely to alter the function of that sequence and, as a result, change the phenotype of the organism in an unexpected fashion. Because two different genetic events would have occurred (disruption of one gene by addition of another), it could be difficult to tease apart the effects of the one event from those of the other.

19. One goal of gene knockout experiments is the determination of a target gene's function by analysis of the phenotype of a null mutant. Phenotype analysis of animals heterozygous for the knockout gene would not be informative because these animals also carry one functional copy of the target gene, which in most cases would mask the effect of the mutant allele. In addition, the knockout gene cannot be faithfully transmitted to offspring at high frequency until the host organism contains the knockout gene in the homozygous state in its sex cells.

20. A change in the phenotype of the organism could indicate successful incorporation of a transgenic construct. A gain of function could be due either to the transgene or to a linked selectable marker gene. A loss of function could be due to insertion of the construct into one of the host organism's genes. Also, in many cases, samples of DNA can be isolated and tested either by PCR amplification or by Southern blot analysis.

21. DNA modification by gene targeting relies on homologous recombination to remove endogenous sequences and replace them with desired exogenous sequences. Gene editing, by contrast, utilizes nucleases to break DNA in a sequence-specific manner, which allows genes to be either removed, corrected, or replaced.

22. One concern that has already been raised is the potential of creating so-called "designer babies," whose genomes are edited for nonmedical reasons, such as to produce physical traits that are seen as desirable to parents. Limiting use of CRISPR-Cas to certain human genes (those that result in medical conditions) could also raise a number of ethical questions, among them: Which diseases "merit" treatment? Who will be charged with making such decisions? Will discriminatory consequences result for untreated individuals? The ethics of genome editing will certainly need to be discussed, and no doubt, guidelines will need to be established.

23. A single guide RNA (sgRNA) is a short RNA molecule that mediates sequence specificity for the Cas9 nuclease. The sgRNA guides Cas9 to the appropriate genomic DNA sequence by binding to a complementary site that is near a PAM sequence. Cas9 cleaves three nucleotides upstream of the PAM site.

24. Repair of CRISPR-Cas9 editing by NHEJ, an error prone pathway, would likely disrupt the function of the target gene. This would be appropriate if the goal were to inactivate a harmful dominant allele in a heterozygous cell. Repair by HDR, when a suitable donor template is provided, allows precise substitutions as well as additions or deletions. This type of repair would be appropriate if the goal were to correct a homozygous recessive mutation.

25. Safety concerns would primarily center on the specificity of the edits, given the possibility of off-target edits and the resulting unwanted genomic changes. Efficiency of editing is also a concern–the induced double-strand breaks might be repaired faithfully by HDR in some cells but by use of the error-prone NHEJ pathway in others, which would raise the possibility that the disease state might persist and the question of whether this treatment be attempted if there is a low chance of success. Another ethical concern is the possibility of inducing heritable changes to embryos. Finally, the question of whether CRISPR-Cas editing should be used to engineer desirable traits is itself an ethical question.

26. One example discussed in the text is the precise modification of the corn *ARGOS8* gene. Scientists removed the weak endogenous promoter and replaced it with a stronger promoter, thereby increasing expression and making the modified corn more drought-tolerant.

27. The creation of either transgenic or knockout animals is a multistep, time-intensive process. By contrast, CRISPR-Cas is both rapid and efficient. In addition, creation of transgenic or knockout animals requires specialized skill sets (such as microinjection into nuclei, transfer of ES cells into blastocyst-stage embryos, transfer of embryos into pseudopregnant foster mothers), whereas CRISPR-Cas is technologically less challenging. Finally, edits by CRISPR-Cas can be very precise, in contrast to other edits, especially those in transgenic animals.

Chapter 18: Genomics, Bioinformatics, and Proteomics

Concept Areas	Corresponding Problems
Genomics Overview	1, 2, 3, 4, 7, 16, 17, 21, 22
Human Genome Project	9, 10, 11, 12, 13, 14
Sequencing	1, 4, 7, 13, 14, 15, 21, 22
Genomic Organization	3, 6, 10, 11, 12
Comparative Genomics	1, 8, 15, 17, 21
Bioinformatics	1, 2, 5, 8, 15, 17, 18, 20
Proteomics	1, 7, 11, 19, 20
Annotation	1, 6, 19
Microarrays	1, 18

Structures and Processes Checklist–Significant items that deserve special attention are identified with a "*".

(Check topic when mastered–provide examples where appropriate–understand the context of each entry)

- **Overview**
  - genomic analysis
  - genomics*
  - bioinformatics*
  - transcriptome analysis*
  - proteomics*
  - synthetic biology*
- **Sequencing Entire Genomes***
  - whole-genome sequencing (WGS)*
  - shotgun sequencing*
  - restriction enzymes*
  - partial digests of DNA
  - alignment*
  - contiguous fragments (contigs)*
  - high-throughput sequencing

- **DNA Sequence Analysis**
  - bioinformatics*
  - GenBank*
  - accession number
  - annotation*
  - BLAST (Basic Local Alignment Search Tool)*
  - query sequence
  - subject sequence
  - identity value*
  - E-value*
  - gene-regulatory regions
  - open reading frame (ORF)*
  - exon*
  - intron*

- splice sites*
- downstream elements
- functional genomics*
- sequence similarity searches
- homologous genes*
- paralog*
- ortholog*
- protein domains*

- **Genome Organization in Humans**
  - Human Genome Project (HGP)*
  - primary goals of HGP*
  - ELSI Program
  - Celera Genomics
  - major features of human genome*
  - reference genome
  - genome is dynamic*
  - approximately 20,000 genes*
  - alternative splicing*
  - functional categories
  - single-nucleotide polymorphisms (SNPs)*
  - copy number variations (CNVs)*
  - HGP on the Internet*

- **The "Omics" Revolution**
  - proteomics
  - metabolomics
  - glycomics
  - toxicogenomics
  - metagenomics

- pharmacogenomics
- transcriptomics
- personal genomics
- personal genome projects (PGPs)
- genome mosaicism
- genomic variation
- pangenome*
- whole-exome sequencing (WES)*
- Encyclopedia of DNA Elements (ENCODE) Project*
- functional elements
- "junk" DNA
- nutrigenomics
- Genome 10K Project*
- stone-age genomics

- **Genomics of Humans and Model Organisms**
  - comparative genomics*
  - more than 23,000 genomes sequenced
  - model organisms
  - sea urchin genome*
  - pseudogenes*
  - intron size correlated with genome size*
  - share about 7000 orthologs with humans
  - human evolution
  - Neanderthal genome*
  - *FOXP2* gene
  - interbreeding

- **Genomics of Environmental Samples**
  - metagenomics
  - environmental genomics*
  - genetic diversity in microbes
  - Human Microbiome Project (HMP)*
  - HMP goals
  - HMP findings
  - no single reference human microbiome
  - Venn diagram
- **Profiles of Expressed Genes**
  - transcriptome analysis
  - transcriptomics*
  - global analysis of gene expression
  - DNA microarray analysis
  - gene chips
  - cDNA
  - expressed sequence tags (ESTs)
  - spots, fields, or features
  - RNA sequencing (RNA-seq)
- **Protein Composition of Cells***
  - proteome*
  - proteomics*
  - proteins as biomarkers*

- Human Proteome Map (HPM)
- two-dimensional gel electrophoresis (2DGE)*
- isoelectric focusing
- sodium dodecyl sulfate polyacrylamide gel electrophoresis (SDS-PAGE)*
- mass spectrometry (MS)
- mass-to-charge (*m/z*) ratio
- *m/z* spectra databases
- matrix-assisted laser desorption ionization (MALDI)
- peptide "fingerprint"
- **Synthetic Biology**
  - minimal genome*
  - synthetic, or artificial, genome
  - "core genes"
  - *Mycoplasma genitalium*
  - synthetic *Mycoplasma mycoides* genome
  - genome transplantation*
  - Human Genome Project-Write (HGP-Write)
  - synthetic biology
  - synthetic biology applications

Answers to Now Solve This

18.1 (a) To annotate a gene, identify gene regulatory sequences found upstream of genes (promoters, enhancers, and silencers), downstream elements (termination sequences), and in-frame triplet nucleotides that are part of the coding region of the gene. In addition, polyadenylation sites as well as 5' and 3' splice sites that are used to distinguish exons from introns are also used in annotation.

(b) Similarity to other annotated sequences often provides insight as to a sequence's function and might serve to substantiate a particular genetic assignment. Direct sequencing of cDNAs from various tissues and developmental stages aids in verification.

(c) The 3141 genes identified on chromosome 1 constitute 15.7 percent of the total number of genes in the human genome (estimated to be 20,000). Since chromosome 1 contains 8 percent of the human genome and almost 16 percent of the genes, it would appear that chromosome 1 is gene rich.

18.2 Structural and chemical factors determine the function of a protein; therefore, it is possible to have several proteins that share a considerable amino acid sequence identity but may not be functionally identical. The *in vivo* function of a protein is determined by secondary and tertiary structures as well as by local surface chemistries in active or functional sites. The nonidentical sequences of the four proteins might have considerable influence on protein folding, overall structure, and, therefore, function. Note that the query sequence matches to different site positions within the target proteins. A number of other factors that suggest different functions include associations with other molecules (cytoplasmic, membrane, or extracellular), chemical nature and position of binding domains, posttranslational modification, and signal sequences.

18.3 Advantages: First, blood is relatively easy to obtain in a pure state, so its components can be analyzed without fear of tissue-site contamination. Second, blood is intimately exposed to virtually all cells of the body and might therefore carry chemical markers to certain abnormal cells. It represents, theoretically, an ideal probe into the human body. **Validation criteria:** When blood is removed from the body, its proteome changes, and those changes are dependent on a number of environmental factors. Thus, what might be a valid diagnostic under one set of conditions might not be so under others. In addition, the serum proteome is subject to change depending on the genetic, physiologic, and environmental states of the patient. Age and sex are additional variables that must be considered. Validation of a plasma proteome for a particular cancer would be strengthened by demonstrating that the stage of development of the cancer correlates with a commensurate change in the proteome in a relatively large, statistically significant pool of patients. As well, the types of changes in the proteome should be reproducible and, at least until complexities are clarified, involve tumorigenic proteins. It would be helpful to have comparisons with archived samples of each individual at a disease-free time.

Solutions to Problems and Discussion Questions

1. (a) Contigs are defined as overlapping segments that collectively form a portion of a chromosome; therefore, if the fragments are known to be contiguous, they are, by definition, part of the same chromosome.

(b) Identification of a protein-coding region is likely if similar sequences are conserved in other species. The presence of various upstream regulatory sequences and downstream elements, splicing donor and acceptor sites (in eukaryotes) in appropriate locations, and a potential open reading frame is further evidence that a sequence encodes a protein.

(c) Comparisons of DNA base sequence data with other organisms indicate conservation of a considerable number of sequences. Because of such conservation, functional relationships are strongly supported. Comparative mutation analyses that indicate similar function add additional support.

(d) Proteomics is the identification and analysis of proteins in cells, tissues, and organisms. Genome annotation provides an estimate of the number of protein coding genes, whereas a number of sophisticated techniques, including electrophoresis, chromatography, and microarrays, indicate the number of proteins actually produced. The finding that there are many more types of proteins than genes in the genome has generated a number of explanations.

(e) The reference genome was considered to be the most accurate sequence available for any organism. For humans, the reference genome consisted of a pool of haploid genomes from many individuals, in an attempt to present the major features shared among populations. Personal genomics, however, have highlighted that such reference genomes underestimate the degree of human genome variations by at least five-fold. Scientists in a number of fields therefore, have chosen to replace a single reference genome by a pangenome, which attempts to represent all variations found in a species.

(f) DNA microarrays provide a platform for hybridization between thousands of known DNA gene probes and sequences that are expressed in the different cell or tissue types of an organism. Comparison of the patterns of hybridization (i.e., which gene probes were hybridized and at what intensity) among all tested cDNAs showed substantial differences, which indicates that whereas some genes are expressed in almost all cells, others show cell- and tissue-specific expression.

2. Your essay should include a description of traditional recombinant DNA technology, which involved cutting and splicing genes, as well as modern methods of synthesizing genes of interest, PCR amplification, microarray analysis, etc.

3. In functional genomics, DNA sequence information is used to predict and understand gene function and to identify gene components such as regulatory elements. In comparative genomics, similarities in DNA (and, therefore, protein) sequences between different organisms are studied. Similarities are used to infer gene function, and differences are used to gain insights into biological, developmental, and evolutionary differences.

4. Whole-genome sequencing involves randomly cutting the genome into numerous smaller segments and determining their sequences. Overlapping sequences are used to identify segments that were once contiguous, eventually producing the entire sequence. Ultimately, entire chromosomes can be sequenced, and the positions of genes, both known and presumptive, precisely mapped. Linkage mapping, by contrast, does not rely on sequence information, but rather on recombination frequencies observed in the progeny of specific crosses. As a result, only relative map distances between known genes can be determined. While this method can also produce a map of an entire chromosome, all distances are relative, and only known genes with detectable phenotypes are mapped.

5. Bioinformatics is the use of computer and mathematics applications to organize, share, and analyze data generated by sequencing. As genomics emerged, bioinformatics became a critical factor in our ability to access and understand the tremendous amounts and varieties of information being made available because it fuses biological data with information technology, mathematics, and statistical analysis. Most applications, such as the identification of informational content in the genome and DNA sequencing, rely on the use of nucleic acid and protein databases.

6. One usually begins to annotate a DNA sequence by comparing it, often using BLAST, to the known sequences already stored in various databases. Similarity to other annotated sequences often provides insight as to a sequence's function. Hallmarks to annotation in both bacteria and eukaryotes are the identification of gene regulatory sequences found upstream (such as promoters) and downstream (termination sequences) of genes, as well as triplet nucleotides that are part of the coding region of the gene. Bacterial genes do not contain a number of the elements found in eukaryotic genes, so their annotation is sometimes less complicated. In eukaryotes, upstream elements would also include enhancers and silencers, and downstream elements would also include a polyadenylation signal sequence (enhancers and silencers are also possible). In addition, 5′ and 3′ splice sites that distinguish exons from introns are also used in annotation.

7. High-throughput technologies reduce the time needed to accomplish labor-intensive tasks from days or weeks to half-days. As a result, more information, often of higher quality, can be gathered. Applied to both genomics and proteomics, high-throughput technologies allow rapid analyses and deployment of genomic information.

8. One initial approach to annotating a DNA sequence is to compare the newly sequenced genomic DNA to the known sequences already stored in various databases. The National Center for Biotechnology Information (NCBI) provides access to BLAST (Basic Local Alignment Search Tool) software that directs searches through databanks of DNA and protein sequences. A segment of DNA can be compared to sequences in major databases such as GenBank to identify matches that align in whole or in part. For example, using a query sequence from mouse chromosome 11, one might find identical or similar sequences in a number of taxa. BLAST will compute an identity value to indicate the degree to which two sequences are similar as well as an "expect" value (E-value, the likelihood that the sequences match by chance), which indicates the level of significance of a match (a value close to 1 indicates the match may be random). BLAST is one of many sequence alignment algorithms (RNA-RNA, protein-protein, etc.) that may sacrifice sensitivity for speed.

9. The main goals of the Human Genome Project are to establish, categorize, and analyze functions for human genes. As stated in the text:

To establish functional categories for all human genes

To analyze genetic variations between humans, including the identification of single-nucleotide polymorphisms (SNPs)

To map and sequence the genomes of several model organisms used in experimental genetics,

including *E. coli, S. cerevisiae, C. elegans, D. melanogaster,* and *M. musculus* (the mouse)

To develop new sequencing technologies, such as high-throughput computer-automated sequencers, to facilitate genome analysis

To disseminate genome information, among both scientists and the general public

10. The human genome is composed of more than 3 billion nucleotides of which about 2 percent code for genes. There appears to be approximately 20,000 protein-coding genes; however, there is still uncertainty as to the total number. Genes are unevenly distributed over chromosomes, with clusters of gene-rich regions separated by gene-poor ones (deserts). Human genes tend to be larger and contain more and larger introns than in invertebrates such as *Drosophila*. It is estimated that at least half of the genes generate products by alternative splicing. The human genome is dynamic, containing an abundance of repetitive sequence scattered throughout.

11. According to the PANTHER database, 5.3 percent of human genes encode transcription factors; 2.4 percent encode cytoskeletal proteins; and 0.3 percent encode transmembrane receptor regulatory/adaptor proteins.

12. Copy number variations (CNVs) are duplications or deletions of large sections of repetitive DNA. Because many CNVs are not directly involved in production of a phenotype, they tend to be isolated from selection and show considerable variation in redundancy. Length variation in such repeats is unique among individuals (except for identical twins). Single-nucleotide polymorphisms also occur frequently in the genome and can be used to distinguish individuals.

13. The PGP provides individual sequences of diploid genomes, and results of such projects indicate that the HGP may underestimate genome variation by as much as fivefold. Genome variation between individuals may be 0.5 percent rather than the 0.1 percent estimated from the HGP. Because the PGP provides sequence information on individuals, fundamental questions about human diversity and evolution may be more answerable.

14. Whole-genome sequencing (the strategy used for the HGP) provides sequences of entire genomes, including noncoding regions, whereas whole-exome sequencing provides sequence information for exons only. Because there are more disease-related variations in the exome than in other regions of the genome, WES is more likely to identify these mutations than is WGS. However, only WGS is able to identify mutations in regulatory regions that lead to disease.

15. Given the speed, efficiency, and recent cost reductions associated with modern sequencing technologies, in 2009, some scientists began to sequence 10,000 (10K) vertebrate genomes. They believed that such a massive pool of sequences would provide insight into genome evolution and speciation, in addition to providing valuable insight to the human genome through comparative genomics.

16. A number of new subdisciplines of molecular biology have been developed and promise to provide the infrastructure for major advances in our understanding of living systems. The following terms identify specific areas within that infrastructure:

- proteomics: proteins in a cell or tissue
- metabolomics: enzymatic pathways
- glycomics: carbohydrates of a cell or tissue
- toxicogenomics: toxic chemicals
- metagenomics: environmental issues
- pharmacogenomics: customized medicine
- transcriptomics: expressed genes

Many other "omics" are likely in the future.

17. Metagenomics is a relatively new discipline that examines the genomes from entire communities of microbes in environmental samples of water, air, and soil. The use of metagenomics can lead to the identification of uncharacterized bacteria and viruses, provide insights regarding the genetic diversity in microbial communities and the interactions between microbes and their environment, and has the potential for identifying genes with novel functions. Virtually every environment on Earth is being sampled in metagenomics projects. Metagenomics is teaching us more about millions of species of microbes, of which only a few thousand have been well characterized. One example is the Human Microbiome Project (HMP), which seeks to understand how this microbiome affects human health.

18. Most DNA microarrays, also known as gene chips, consist of a glass slide that is coated, using a robotic system, with thousands of spots, each containing multiple copies of a different single-stranded DNA (probes). Some microarrays use

sequences of expressed sequenced tags or DNA sequences that are complementary to gene transcripts as probes. A single microarray can have as many as 20,000 different spots of DNA (or as many as 1 million for exon-specific arrays), each containing a unique sequence. Researchers use microarrays to compare patterns of gene expression in tissues under different conditions or to compare gene expression patterns in normal and diseased tissues. In addition, microarrays can be used to identify pathogens.

19. Increased protein production from approximately 20,000 genes is probably related to alternative splicing and various posttranslational processing schemes. In addition, a particular DNA segment may be read in a variety of ways and in both directions.

20. (a) More than 290,000 nonredundant peptides were identified from multiple organs, tissues, and cell types from clinically healthy individuals.

(b) Seven fetal tissues were used.

(c) A wide variety of searches can be performed.

21. Any time a DNA sequence is conserved in other species, it is likely that that sequence has an influence on similar phenotypes. The higher the number of species with the conserved sequence, the higher the likelihood of determining its function. Coupled with mutation analysis and physical mapping, comparative genomics provides a powerful method for linking DNA sequences with complex human diseases.

22. (a) The strength of WES is that one might get lucky and identify a coding issue in a gene that has relevance to the patient's condition. However, there are several weaknesses to this approach. Given the multitude of genetic variations known to exist, using this approach might be akin to looking for a needle in a haystack. In addition, many important regulatory and structural components in the genome are outside the exon pool and would not be detected by this method.

(b) Depending on the symptoms and the nature of the disorder, examination of the mitochondrial genome (which is highly variable between individuals) might be advisable because the list of human conditions known to involve mitochondrial defects is growing. However, the high degree of genetic variability of mtDNA might make identification of meaningful differences difficult.

Chapter 19: The Genetics of Cancer

Concept Areas	Corresponding Problems
Cancer Origins	1, 2, 13, 16, 17, 18, 19, 23, 24, 25, 26, 27
Cancer Biology	1, 6, 16, 19, 21, 23, 24, 25
Inherited Cancer Predisposition	7, 22, 26, 27
Repair Mechanisms	1, 12, 18
Cell-Cycle Dynamics	3, 4, 5, 6, 11, 21
Cell-Cycle Mechanisms	4, 5, 11, 12, 18
Cancer and the Environment	17, 20, 21
Apoptosis	8, 18, 21
Tumor Suppressors and Oncogenes	9, 10, 11, 12, 13, 14, 15, 22, 26, 27
Chromosome Structure	2, 15, 23

Structures and Processes Checklist–Significant items that deserve special attention are identified with a "*".

(Check topic when mastered–provide examples where appropriate–understand the context of each entry)

- **Overview**

  - numerous abnormal gene products

- **Cancer Is a Genetic Disease**

  - genomic alterations*

  - predominantly somatic cell mutations

  - accumulation of mutations

  - proliferation*

  - metastasis*

  - benign tumor

  - metastases

  - malignant tumor

  - clonal*

  - Burkitt lymphoma

  - reciprocal translocations

  - cancer subclones

  - driver mutations*

  - passenger mutations*

  - cancer stem cells

  - cancer stem cell hypothesis*

  - random, or stochastic, model

  - multiple mutations*

  - multistep process*

  - carcinogen*

  - tumorigenesis

  - clonal expansion

  - adenoma, or polyp

  - *adenomatous polyposis coli (APC)* gene

  - *KRAS* gene

  - carcinoma

  - *TP53, PI3K, TGF-β*

- **Cancer and Genomic Stability***
  - mutator phenotype*
  - genomic instability
  - chronic myelogenous leukemia (CML)*
  - Philadelphia chromosome
  - reciprocal translocation*
  - BCR-ABL protein*
  - protein kinase
  - defective DNA repair*
  - xeroderma pigmentosum (XP)
  - hereditary nonpolyposis colorectal cancer (HNPCC)*
  - epigenetics*
  - chromatin modifications*
  - altered DNA methylation*
  - histone modifications*
- **Cancer and Cell-Cycle Regulation***
  - differentiated cells*
  - cell cycle
  - G1, S, G2, M
  - G0
  - signal transduction*
  - G1/S checkpoint*
  - G2/M checkpoint*
  - M checkpoint*
  - cyclins*
  - cyclin-dependent kinases (CDKs)*
  - CDK/cyclin complex
  - apoptosis, or programmed cell death*
- caspases*
- **Cancer-Related Genes***
  - proto-oncogene
  - oncogene*
  - tumor-suppressor genes*
  - *ras* gene family*
  - inactive/active state
  - GDP/GTP bound
  - *TP53* gene*
  - p53 protein*
  - MDM2*
  - p21 protein
  - CDK4/cyclin D1 complex
- **Cancer Cells Metastasize***
  - extracellular matrix*
  - basal lamina
  - E-cadherin glycoprotein
  - metalloproteinases*
  - tissue inhibitors of metalloproteinases (TIMPs)*
- **Inherited Predisposition***
  - loss of heterozygosity*
  - cancer pre-disposition genes
  - familial adenomatous polyposis (FAP)*
  - *APC* heterozygosity*
  - polyp formation
- **Viruses and Environmental Agents***
  - chemicals
  - aflatoxin
  - nitrosamines

- metabolism
- radiation
- radon gas
- dietary factors

- pollutants
- tobacco smoke
- some viruses

Answers to Now Solve This

19.1 Being able to distinguish leukemic cells from healthy cells allows not only the design of a therapy and the subsequent targeting of a specific cell population, but also the quantification of responses to that therapy. One therapeutic approach is to inactivate the BCR-ABL protein. It is known that the fusion protein acts as unregulated protein kinase, which tells the cells to proliferate even though there is no external signal calling for them to do so. As a fusion protein, BCR-ABL has a unique structure. It is theoretically possible, then, that an inhibitor could be synthesized that is specific to the fusion protein. In other words, one could create a drug that would "turn off" the BCR-ABL protein without affecting the function any of the other protein kinases. This is exactly what scientists at Ciba-Geigy (now Novartis) did in the production of Gleevec (see link provided in the question). An alternative therapeutic approach might be to develop an immunotherapy, based on the uniqueness of the BCR-ABL protein.

19.2 *TP53* is a tumor suppressor gene that encodes a protein to protect cells from multiplying with damaged DNA. It is present in its mutant state in more than 50 percent of all tumors. *TP53* mediates the immediate control of a critical and universal cell-cycle checkpoint, and its action is not limited to specific cell types. As a result, mutation of this gene will influence a wide range of cell types and give rise to a diversity of tumors.

19.3 Cancer is a complex alteration in normal cell-cycle controls. Even if a major "cancer-causing" gene is transmitted, other genes, often new mutations, are usually necessary in order to drive a cell toward tumor formation. Mutations of genes that encode DNA repair proteins will make the individual particularly susceptible (the mutator phenotype). Full expression of the cancer phenotype is likely to be the result of interplay among a variety of genes and therefore likely to show variable penetrance and expressivity.

19.4 Unfortunately, it is common to spend enormous amounts of money dealing with diseases after they occur rather than concentrating on disease prevention. Too often, pressure from special interest groups or lack of political will retards advances in education and prevention. Obviously, it is less expensive, in terms of both human suffering and money, to seek preventive measures for as many diseases as possible. However, having gained some understanding of the mechanisms of disease, in this case, cancer, it must also be stated that no matter what preventive measures are taken, it will be impossible to completely eliminate disease from the human population. It is extremely important, however, that we increase efforts to educate and protect the human population from as many hazardous environmental agents as possible. A balanced, multipronged approach seems appropriate.

Chapter 19 The Genetics of Cancer

Solutions to Problems and Discussion Questions

1. (a) The clonal origin of cancer cells in a given cancer is supported by findings that mutations, chromosomal or otherwise, are of the same type in all cancerous cells.

(b) The progressive, time- and age-dependent development of tumorigenesis, coupled with the relatively low cancer rate compared to the mutation rate, argues for a multistep mutational model for cancer.

(c) The mutator phenotype, thought by some to be caused by defective DNA repair mechanisms, is characteristic of cancer cells. Numerous cancers, exemplified by xeroderma pigmentosum and hereditary nonpolyposis colorectal cancer, are caused by defective DNA repair systems.

2. Your essay should describe the general influence of genetics in cancer. Epigenetic factors can alter gene expression, making it likely that changes in such factors could cause cancer.

3. Signal transduction is the process by which signals from the external environment are received by cells and then transmitted to the nucleus. These signals can call for the cell to reenter the cell cycle and ultimately divide (proliferation). Cancer cells often have defective signal transduction pathways that continuously call for proliferation.

4. The major regulatory points of the cell cycle include the following:

- late G1 (G1/S)
- the border between G2 and mitosis (G2/M)
- mitosis (M)

5. Kinases regulate other proteins by adding phosphate groups. Cyclins bind to a class of kinases, the cyclin dependent kinases (or cdks), switching them on and off. For example, when cyclin D binds to CDK4, the complex acts to move cells from G1 to S. At the G2/mitosis border, another CDK/cyclin complex (CDK1/cyclin B) forms, and the resulting phosphorylation brings about a series of changes in the nuclear membrane, cytoskeleton, and chromosomes.

6. Differentiated cells are specialized for specific functions, whereas cancer cells tend to be less specialized. In addition, differentiated cells can enter a G0 phase of the cell cycle and remain quiescent indefinitely. Although these cells do not usually divide, some are able to do so if stimulated by extracellular signals, such as growth factors. Cancer cells, by contrast, are not only able to self-renew, they are unable to enter G0 and, instead, cycle continuously.

7. To say that a particular trait is inherited conveys the assumption that when a particular genotype is present, it will be revealed in the phenotype. For instance, albinism is inherited in such a way that individuals who are homozygous recessive express albinism. When one discusses an inherited predisposition, one usually refers to situations in which a particular phenotype is expressed in families in some consistent pattern. Cancer predisposition genes are mutations in the germ line, often of proto-oncogenes or tumor-suppressor genes. Although the mutation is, itself, insufficient to cause cancer, inheritance of the gene does increase the risk of developing cancer. In individuals who carry a cancer predisposition gene, another somatic mutation or loss of heterozygosity might trigger tumor development and, possibly, malignancy.

8. Apoptosis, or programmed cell death, is a genetically controlled process that leads to death of a cell. It is a natural process involved in morphogenesis and a protective mechanism against cancer formation. During apoptosis, nuclear DNA becomes fragmented, cellular structures are disrupted, and the cells are dissolved. Caspases are involved in the initiation and progress of apoptosis.

9. A tumor-suppressor gene product normally functions to regulate the cell cycle or to initiate apoptosis. When tumor-suppressor proteins are inactive, cell-cycle checkpoints are ignored, and/or apoptosis is not triggered. As a result, mutations in other genes can accumulate, and tumors or cancer might develop. From an evolutionary standpoint, it makes sense that sufficient quantities of this gene product are made from just one of the two alleles present to provide normal function (haplosufficiency).

10. Under normal conditions, the p53 protein is bound by another protein, MDM2, which keeps p53 in an inactive state. MDM2 not only marks p53 for degradation, it also blocks the p53 transcription activation domain and prevents posttranslational modifications that activate p53. Upon DNA damage or cellular stress, MDM2 dissociates from p53, which both stabilizes the protein and exposes the transcription activation domain. Increases in acetylation and phosphorylation of p53 also contribute to increases in the protein's activity.

11. The p53 protein is a transcriptional regulator. At the G1/S checkpoint, activated p53 acts to increase transcription of the p21 protein which, in turn, prevents the interaction between cyclin D and CDK4. As a result, the cell cycle is arrested before S phase. Similarly, p53 can also regulate transcription of the appropriate genes during S phase and at the G2/M checkpoint, to allow cells sufficient time to replicate DNA or repair DNA damage.

12. At the G2/M checkpoint, physiological conditions in the cell are monitored prior to mitosis. If DNA replication or repair of any DNA damage has not been completed, the cell cycle arrests until these processes are complete. Activated p53 protein regulates expression of genes that retard the progress of DNA replication and that prevent cells from passing the G2/M checkpoint. This allows time for DNA damage to be repaired.

13. Oncogenes are genes that induce or maintain the uncontrolled cellular proliferation associated with cancer. They are mutant forms of proto-oncogenes, which normally function to regulate cell division. Oncogenes may be formed through point mutations, gene amplification, translocations, repositioning of regulatory sequences, or other mechanisms.

14. Mutations that produce oncogenes act in a dominant capacity. Proto-oncogenes normally function to promote or maintain cell division. In the mutant state (oncogenes), they induce or maintain uncontrolled cell division; that is, there is a gain of function. Generally, this gain of function takes the form of increased or abnormally continuous gene output. On the other hand, mutations in tumor-suppressor genes, which function to halt passage through the cell cycle, are generally attributed to loss of function. When such genes are mutant, they have lost their capacity to halt the cell cycle. Such mutations are generally recessive.

15. A reciprocal translocation between chromosomes 9 and 22 is responsible for the generation of the Philadelphia chromosome. Genetic mapping established that certain genes were combined to form a hybrid oncogene (*BCR-ABL*), which encodes a fusion protein that has been implicated in the formation of chronic myelogenous leukemia.

16. Driver mutations are those mutations in a tumor cell that confer a growth advantage upon that cell. Passenger mutations constitute all the remaining mutations in a tumor cell, which do not directly induce a cancerous state. However, any passenger mutation that provides a growth advantage after a change in environmental conditions will become a driver mutation.

17. Significant environmental agents include tobacco smoke, infection by certain viruses, a variety of chemicals, metabolic byproducts, radiation, and diet. For a comprehensive list, review Section 19.7 in the text.

18. Normal cells are often capable of withstanding mutational assault because they have checkpoints and DNA repair mechanisms in place. Cases of severe damage may lead to apoptosis. When such mechanisms fail, cancer may be a result. Through mutation, such protective mechanisms are compromised in cancer cells, and as a result, they show higher-than-normal rates of mutation, chromosomal abnormalities, and genomic instability.

19. Loss of heterozygosity occurs when the normal allele is rendered nonfunctional in a heterozygote. If the normal gene is a tumor suppressor, then its loss may expose a gene that can cause cancer.

20. Certain environmental agents such as chemicals and X rays cause DNA damage that can lead to mutations. DNA repair mechanisms can correct most of the damage, but some might persist. If these mutations affect cell-cycle checkpoint controls, they can lead to cancer.

21. Radiotherapy is often administered externally or internally to damage the cell-cycle machinery, preferentially targeting actively dividing cells. If the damage is extensive, apoptosis or other forms of cell death may be triggered, thus shrinking the cancer. This therapy may be completely or only partially effective. Side effects are expected, since the treatment targets proliferating cells but does not distinguish between normal and cancerous cells. Some damage to normal cells can be mitigated by their DNA repair systems.

22. No, she will still have the same risk as the general female population (about 12 percent). In addition, it is possible that genetic tests will not detect all breast cancer mutations.

23. The cancer stem cell hypothesis proposes that only a limited number of cells in a tumor proliferate. Those that do are stem cells–undifferentiated cells that give rise to two populations of daughter cells; one will differentiate and the other remains a stem cell and continues to proliferate. This contrasts with the stochastic model in which every tumor cell is considered to have the capacity to divide and form a new tumor.

24. A benign tumor is a mass of proliferating cells that is usually localized to a given anatomical site. Such tumors can usually be removed surgically. Malignant tumors are also multicellular masses, but not all the cells are contained. Some cells are able to break away, invade other tissues, and form tumors at one or more secondary sites. Malignant tumors are more difficult to treat and can be much more life-threatening than benign tumors.

25. Metastasis, the process by which malignancies spread to other tissues, occurs when a cancer cell invades another tissue. Tissues are surrounded by the extracellular matrix, composed of proteins and carbohydrates, which serves as a scaffold for growth and inhibits cell migration. Therefore, for tissue invasion to occur, the malignant cell must digest the extracellular matrix, which requires a protease. A mutation in a protease-encoding gene would likely render it unresponsive to regulation.

26. As with many forms of cancer, a single genetic alteration is not the only requirement. The authors (Bose et al.) state, "but only infrequently do the cells acquire the additional changes necessary to produce leukemia in humans." It is possible that the cells that produce these transcripts are extremely low in number (the PCR detection method used was very sensitive) and are unable to establish themselves as key stem cells for clonal expansion, which is necessary for cancer formation. Finally, it is also possible that the transcripts produced do not result in a functional fusion protein.

27. (a) The most straightforward way to determine whether the cells carry a normal copy of the *RB1* gene is sequencing. Sequence the normal *RB1* allele from the cDNA clone. Using this sequence, design PCR primers to amplify the *RB1* alleles from the osteosarcoma culture cells and sequence the amplified products. Comparison of the sequences should reveal any differences.

Alternatively, using NGS methods, sequence the genome of the osteosarcoma cells, then use bioinformatic analysis to search for sequences that match the known *RB1* sequence. If the cells contain one normal copy, this should be detected.

(b) Make antibodies to pRB from the noncancerous cells and test these antibodies for reactivity against proteins from the cancerous cell lines. A pRB-antibody reaction would indicate that the pRB protein is made.

Alternatively, use MALDI to develop a protein fingerprint of the osteosarcoma cells and look for an *m/z* ratio characteristic of pRB.

(c) To determine whether addition of a normal *RB1* gene will change the cancer-causing potential of osteosarcoma cells, transfer the cloned normal *RB1* gene into the cells by transformation. Next, introduce the transformed cells into the cancer-prone mice to determine whether their cancer-causing potential had been altered.

Chapter 20: Quantitative Genetics and Multifactorial Traits

Concept Areas	Corresponding Problems
Phenotypic Expression	1, 4, 5, 6, 7, 10, 16, 21
Continuous Variation and Polygenes	1, 2, 3, 4, 5, 6, 7, 10, 11, 12, 21
Genetic Basis	1, 2, 3, 4, 5, 6, 7
Heritability	1, 3, 8, 9, 13, 14, 15, 16, 17, 18, 19, 20
Statistics	12, 16
Twin Studies	1, 3, 8, 9

Structures and Processes Checklist–Significant items that deserve special attention are identified with a "*".

(Check topic when mastered–provide examples where appropriate–understand the context of each entry)

- **Overview**

  - continuous variation*

  - quantitative inheritance*

  - polygenic

  - polygenes*

  - multifactorial, or complex traits

- **Quantitative Traits and Mendelian Inheritance**

  - multiple-factor, or multiple-gene hypothesis*

  - cumulative or quantitative contribution

  - additive allele*

  - nonadditive allele*

  - calculate number of polygenes*

  - $1/4^n$

  - $(2n + 1)$

- **Statistical Analysis**

  - sample

- normal distribution*

- central tendency*

- mean ($\bar{X}$)*

- $\bar{X} = \dfrac{\sum X_i}{n}$

- variance (s^2)*

- $s^2 = \dfrac{\sum\left(X_i - \bar{X}\right)^2}{n-1}$

- standard deviation (s)*

- $s = \sqrt{s^2}$

- standard error of the mean ($S_{\bar{X}}$)*

- $S_{\bar{X}} = \dfrac{s}{\sqrt{n}}$

- covariance (cov_{XY})

- $\text{cov}_{XY} = \dfrac{\sum\left[(X_i - \bar{X})(Y_i - \bar{Y})\right]}{n-1}$

- correlation coefficient (r)

- $r = \dfrac{\mathrm{cov}_{XY}}{S_X S_Y}$

- **Genetic Contribution to Variability***

  - heritability*

  - phenotypic variance (V_P)*

  - genotypic variance (V_G)*

  - environmental variance (V_E)*

  - genotype-by-environment variance ($V_{G \times E}$)*

  - $V_P = V_G + V_E + V_{G \times E}$

  - broad-sense heritability (H^2)*

  - $H^2 = \dfrac{V_G}{V_P}$

  - narrow-sense heritability (h^2)*

  - additive variance (V_A)

  - dominance variance (V_D)

  - interactive variance (V_I)

  - $V_G = V_A + V_D + V_I$

  - $h^2 = \dfrac{V_A}{V_P}$

  - $h^2 = \dfrac{V_A}{V_E + V_A + V_D}$

  - artificial selection

  - selection response (R)*

  - $R = M2 - M$

  - selection differential (S)

  - $S = M1 - M$

- $h^2 = \dfrac{R}{S}$

- limitations of heritability studies

- **Twin Studies***

  - monozygotic (MZ), or identical, twins*

  - dizygotic (DZ), or fraternal, twins*

  - concordant*

  - discordant*

  - differences between concordance values of MZ and DZ

  - additive model

  - genome-wide association studies (GWAS)

  - limitations of twin studies*

  - copy number variation (CNV)

  - somatic mosaicism

  - epigenetics*

  - DNA methylation patterns

- **Studying Multifactorial Phenotypes***

  - quantitative trait locus (QTL)

  - QTL mapping*

  - QTL mapping population*

  - chromosome-specific DNA markers*

  - cosegregate

  - expression QTLs (eQTLs)

Answers to Now Solve This

20.1 **(a)** Because approximately 1/256 of the F_2 plants are 20 cm and approximately 1/256 are 40 cm, there must be four gene pairs $(1/4^4 = 1/256)$ involved in determining flower size.

(b) The back cross is $AaBbCcDd \times AABBCCDD$, and the frequency distribution in the backcross would be:

1/16	=	40 cm
4/16	=	37.5 cm
6/16	=	35 cm
4/16	=	32.5 cm
1/16	=	30 cm

20.2 **(a)** Use the equations provided in both the text chapter and the checklist above to calculate the following values:

The mean for each is

   sheep fiber length: 7.7 cm   *fleece weight*: 6.4 kg

The variance for each is

   sheep fiber length: 6.097   *fleece weight*: 3.12

The standard deviation for each is

   sheep fiber length: 2.469   *fleece weight*: 1.766

(b) The covariance for the two traits is 30.36/7, or 4.34.

(c) The correlation coefficient is +0.998.

(d) The correlation coefficient indicates that there is a very high correlation between fleece weight and fiber length, and it is likely that this correlation is not by chance. Even though correlation does not mean cause and effect, it would seem logical that as you increased fiber length, you would also increase fleece weight. It is probably safe to assume that the increase in fleece weight is directly related to an increase in fiber length.

20.3 Compare the expression of traits in monozygotic and dizygotic twins. A higher concordance value for monozygotic twins indicates a significant genetic component for a given trait. Notice that for traits including blood type, eye color, and mental retardation, there is a fairly substantial difference between MZ and DZ groups. However, for measles and handedness, the difference is not as large, indicating the environment has a greater role. Hair color has a substantial genetic component, as do idiopathic epilepsy, schizophrenia, diabetes, allergies, cleft lip, and club foot. The genetic component to mammary cancer is present but minimal according to these data.

Chapter 20 Quantitative Genetics and Multifactorial Traits

Solutions to Problems and Discussion Questions

1. (a) If the ratio of F_2 individuals resembling either of the two extreme P_1 phenotypes can be determined, then the number of polygenes involved in a polygenic trait can often be estimated by solving for n in the formula $1/4^n$.

It is also possible to estimate the number of polygenes using the $(2n + 1)$ rule, where $(2n + 1)$ is the number of possible phenotypes, and n equals the number of additive loci.

(b) The multiple-factor hypothesis was originally based on experiments involving pigmentation in wheat. The results showed that a number of additive alleles acting in Mendelian fashion could explain continuous variation.

(c) When a number of parameters are known, environmental impact on a quantitatively inherited trait is often assessed by heritability estimates (broad and narrow sense). Use of highly inbred strains of plants and animals reared under varying conditions and twin studies in humans are helpful in determining the environmental impact on specific traits.

(d) Differences in inherited disease states indicate that gene copy number variation and epigenetics alter the genotypes of all individuals, including monozygotic twins.

2. Your essay should include a description of various ratios typical of Mendelian genetics as compared with the more blending, continuously varying expressions of Neomendelian modes of inheritance. It should contrast discontinuous inheritance and continuous patterns.

3. (a) *Polygenes* are genes involved in determining continuously varying or multiple-factor traits. *Polygenic* refers to traits that result from the input of many genes.

(b) *Additive alleles* are those alleles that account for the hereditary influence on the phenotype in an additive way.

(c) *Monozygotic twins* are derived from a single fertilized egg and are thus genetically identical to each other at the start of their lives. They provide a method for determining the influence of genetics and environment on certain traits. *Dizygotic twins* arise from two eggs, each fertilized by a separate sperm cell. They have the same genetic relationship as siblings.

The role of genetics and the role of the environment can be studied by comparing the expression of traits in monozygotic and dizygotic twins, raised together versus apart. A higher concordance value for monozygotic twins as compared with the value for dizygotic twins indicates a significant genetic component for a given trait.

(d) *Heritability* is a measure of the degree to which the phenotypic variation of a given trait is due to genetic factors within a certain population in a particular environment. A high heritability indicates that genetic factors are major contributors to phenotypic variation, whereas environmental factors have little impact.

(e) *QTL* stands for quantitative trait locus, a chromosomal region that contains one or more genes that contribute to a quantitative trait.

4. There are two ways to solve this. (1) Determine the ratio of F_2 individuals expressing either extreme phenotype, then apply the formula $1/4^n$ to determine the number of polygenes (n). (2) Use the number of phenotypic categories to calculate the number of polygenes (n) by applying the formula $(2n + 1)$.

(a) Because a dihybrid result has been identified, two loci are involved in the production of color. Two alleles are at each locus for a total of four alleles.

(b, c) Because the description of color (red, medium red, and so on) gives us no indication of a *quantity* of color in any form of units, we are not able to quantify a unit amount for each change in color. We *can* say that each additive allele provides an equal unit amount to the phenotype, and the colors differ from each other by multiples of that unit amount. The number of additive alleles needed to produce each phenotype follows:

1/16	= dark red	= 4 alleles	*AABB*
4/16	= medium-dark red	= 3 alleles	2 *AABb*
			2 *AaBB*
6/16	= medium red	= 2 alleles	*AAbb*
			4 *AaBb*
			aaBB
4/16	= light red	= 1 allele	2 *aaBb*
			2 *Aabb*
1/16	= white	= 0 alleles	*aabb*

(d) F_1 = all light red
F_2 = 1/4 medium red
2/4 light red
1/4 white

5. (a) It is *possible* that two parents of moderate height can produce offspring who are much taller or shorter than either parent because segregation can produce a variety of gametes as follows:

$$rrSsTtuu \quad \times \quad RrSsTtUu$$
(moderate)   (moderate)

Offspring from this cross can range from very tall *RrSSTTUu* (14 "tall" units) to very short *rrssttuu* (8 short units).

(b) If the individual with a minimum height, *rrssttuu*, is married to an individual of intermediate height, *RrSsTtUu*, the offspring can be no taller than the height of the tallest parent. Notice that there is no way of having more than four fully additive alleles in the offspring.

6. (a) The data indicate that height is determined by quantitative trait loci.

(b) About $1/250$ F_2 plants exhibit each of the extreme phenotypes, a value that is quite close to $1/256$. Use the formula $1/4^n$ to calculate that four gene pairs involved.

(c) If there are four gene pairs, there are nine $(2n + 1)$ phenotypic categories and eight increments between these categories. Because there is a difference of 24 cm between the extremes, $24\text{ cm}/8 = 3$ cm for each increment (each of the additive alleles).

(d) The shortest extreme, representing the completely recessive genotype (*aabbccdd*), is 12 cm tall and each parental plant is 24 cm tall. If each additive (uppercase) allele contributes 3 cm to plant height, each parental plant must have four additive alleles. Given the uniformity of the F_1 plants, we can conclude that each parental plant is homozygous. Furthermore, the size distribution in the F_2 generation [particularly the presence of 12-cm (*aabbccdd*) and 36-cm (*AABBCCDD*) plants] indicates that all gene pairs in the F_1 plants are heterozygous (*AaBbCcDd*) and independently assorting. Therefore, the parental plants must be homozygous dominant in *different* gene pairs. There are many possible sets of parents that would fit this description. An example is:

$$AABBccdd \quad \times \quad aabbCCDD$$

(e) Two additive alleles are needed for a height of 18 cm. There are many possibilities, with three shown, as follows:

AAbbccdd,
AaBbccdd,
aaBbCcdd, and so on.

Likewise, any plant with seven additive alleles will be 33 cm tall:

AABBCCDd,
AABBCcDD,
AABbCCDD, are three examples.

7. (a) There is a fairly continuous range of "quantitative" phenotypes in the F_2 and an F_1 that is between the phenotypes of the two parents; therefore, one can conclude that this is probably the result of several gene pairs acting in an additive fashion. Because the extreme phenotypes (6 cm and 30 cm) each represent $1/64$ of the total, it is likely that there are three gene pairs in this cross ($1/64 = 1/4^3$). In addition, there are seven categories of phenotypes, which fits the relationship $2n + 1 = 7$, giving the number of gene pairs (n) as 3. The genotypes of the parents would be combinations of alleles that would produce a 6-cm (*aabbcc*) tail and a 30-cm (*AABBCC*) tail, whereas the 18-cm offspring would have a genotype of *AaBbCc*.

(b) A mating of an *AaBbCc* (for example) pig with the 6-cm *aabbcc* pig would result in the following offspring:

Gametes (18-cm tail)	Gamete (6-cm tail)	Offspring
ABC		AaBbCc (18 cm)
ABc		AaBbcc (14 cm)
AbC		AabbCc (14 cm)
Abc	abc	Aabbcc (10 cm)
aBC		aaBbCc (14 cm)
aBc		aaBbcc (10 cm)
abC		aabbCc (10 cm)
abc		aabbcc (6 cm)

In this example, a 1:3:3:1 ratio is the result. However, had a different 18-cm tailed pig been selected, a different ratio would occur:

$$AABbcc \quad \times \quad aabbcc$$

Gametes (18-cm tail)	Gamete (6-cm tail)	Offspring
ABc	abc	AaBbcc (14 cm)
Abc		Aabbcc (10 cm)

8. For height, notice that average differences between MZ twins reared together (1.7 cm) and those MZ twins reared apart (1.8 cm) are similar (meaning little environmental influence) and considerably less than differences of DZ twins (4.4 cm) or sibs (4.5) reared together. These data indicate that genetics plays a major role in determining height.

However, for weight, notice that MZ twins reared together have a much smaller (1.9-kg) difference than MZ twins reared apart, indicating that the environment has a considerable impact on weight. By comparing the weight differences of MZ twins reared apart with DZ twins and sibs reared together, one can conclude that the environment has more of an influence on weight than does genetics.

For ridge count, the differences between MZ twins reared together and those reared apart are small. Overall, for the data presented, ridge count and height appear to have the highest heritability values.

9. Comparison of phenotypic variances between monozygotic and dizygotic traits provides an estimate of broad-sense heritability (H^2).

10. Many traits, especially those we view as quantitative, are likely to be determined by a polygenic mode with possible environmental influences. The following are some common examples: height, general body structure, skin color, and perhaps most common behavioral traits, including intelligence.

11. The solution to these types of problems rests on determining the ratio of individuals expressing the extreme phenotype to the total number of individuals. In this case the ratios are 1:1014 (or 1:338) and 5:1014 (or about 1:203), both of which are closer to 1:256 ($1:4^4$) than to either 1/64 ($1:4^3$) or 1:1024 ($1/:4^5$). Therefore, these data indicate that four gene pairs influence size in these guinea pigs.

12. At first glance, this problem may appear repetitive or tedious to solve; however, it can be simplified.

(a) The mean is computed by adding the measurements of all of the individuals, then dividing by the total number of individuals. In this case, there are 760 corn plants. To keep from having to add 760 numbers, multiply each height group by the number of individuals in each group. Add all the products, then divide by n, which is 760. This gives a value for the mean of 140 cm.

(b) The formula for variance as given both in the text and in the checklist above is

$$s^2 = \frac{\Sigma\left(X_i - \bar{X}\right)^2}{n-1}$$

To avoid adding the same numbers repeatedly for each height category, you can multiply each squared difference by the number of plants in that category, then perform the summation step.

For the first group (100 cm), we would have

$$(100 - 140)^2 \times 20 = 32,000$$

The remaining groups are as follows:

$$(110 - 140)^2 \times 60 = 54,000$$
$$(120 - 140)^2 \times 90 = 36,000$$
$$(130 - 140)^2 \times 130 = 13,000$$
$$(140 - 140)^2 \times 180 = 0$$
$$(150 - 140)^2 \times 120 = 12,000$$
$$(160 - 140)^2 \times 70 = 28,000$$
$$(170 - 140)^2 \times 50 = 45,000$$
$$\underline{(180 - 140)^2 \times 40 = 64,000}$$

Total	284,000

Determine the variance by dividing this sum by $(n - 1)$, which gives: 284,000/759.

Therefore, the variance is $s^2 = 374.18$

(c) The *standard deviation* is the square root of the variance, or 19.34.

(d) The *standard error* of the mean is the standard deviation divided by the square root of n, or about 0.70. The plot approximates a normal distribution. Variation is continuous.

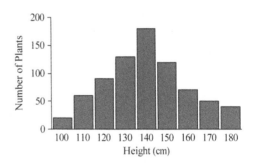

13. **(a)** Using the following equations,

$$H^2 = \frac{V_G}{V_P} \quad \text{and} \quad h^2 = \frac{V_A}{V_P}$$

H^2 and h^2 can be calculated as follows.

For back fat:

Broad-sense heritability = H^2 = 12.2/30.6 = 0.398
Narrow-sense heritability = h^2 = 8.44/30.6 = 0.276

For body length:

Broad-sense heritability = H^2 = 26.4/52.4 = 0.504
Narrow-sense heritability = h^2 = 11.7/52.4 = 0.223

(b) For a trait that is quantitatively measured, the relative importance of genetic *versus* environmental factors may be formally assessed by examining the heritability index (H^2 or broad heritability). In animal and plant breeding, a measure of potential response to selection based on additive variance and dominance variance is termed narrow-sense heritability (h^2). A relatively high narrow-sense heritability is a prediction of the impact selection may have in altering an initial randomly breeding population. Therefore, of the two traits, selection for back fat would produce more response.

14. The formula for estimating heritability is

$$H^2 = {V_G}\Big/{V_P}$$

where V_G and V_P are the genetic and phenotypic components of variation, respectively. The main issue in this question is obtaining some estimate of two components of phenotypic variation: genetic and environmental. V_P is the combination of genetic and environmental variance. Because the two parental strains are inbred, they are assumed to be homozygous, and the variances of 4.2 and 3.8 are considered to be the result of environmental influences. The average of these two values is 4.0. The F_1 is also genetically homogeneous and gives us an additional estimation of the environmental factors.

By averaging this value with that of the parents,

[(4.0 + 5.6)/2 = 4.8]

we obtain a relatively good idea of environmental impact on the phenotype. The phenotypic variance in the F_2 is the sum of the genetic (V_G) and environmental (V_E) components. We have estimated the environmental input as 4.8, so 10.3 (V_P) minus 4.8 gives us an estimate of (V_G), which is 5.5. Heritability then becomes 5.5/10.3 or 0.53. This value, when viewed in percentage form, indicates that about 53 percent of the variation in plant height is due to genetic influences.

15. (a) For vitamin A:

$$h_A^2 = {V_A}\Big/{V_P} = \frac{V_A}{(V_E + V_A + V_D)} = 0.097$$

For cholesterol: $h_A^2 = 0.223$

(b) Cholesterol content should be influenced to a greater extent by selection.

16. Given that both narrow-sense heritability values are relatively high, it is likely that a farmer would be able to alter both milk protein content and butterfat by selection. The value of 0.91 for the correlation coefficient between protein content and butterfat suggests that if one selects for butterfat, protein content will increase. However, correlation coefficients describe the extent to which variation in one quantitative trait is associated with variation in another and do not reveal the underlying causes of such variation. Assuming that these dairy cows had been selected for high butterfat in the past and increased protein content followed that selection (for butterfat), it is likely that selection for butterfat would continue to correlate with increased protein content. However, there may well be a point where physiological circumstances change and selection for high butterfat may be at the expense of protein content.

17. h^2 = (7.5 – 8.5/6.0 – 8.5) = 0.4

(realized heritability)

18. Given the realized heritability value of 0.4, it is unlikely that selection experiments would cause a rapid and/or significant response to selection. A minor response might result from intense selection.

19. h^2 = 0.3 = ($M2$ – 60/80 – 60)

$M2$ = 66 grams

20. Because the rice plants are genetically identical, V_G is zero and $H^2 = V_G/V_P$ = zero. Broad-sense heritability is a measure in which the phenotypic variance is due to genetic factors. In this case, with genetically identical plants, H^2 is zero, and the variance observed in grain yield is due to the environment. Selection would not be effective in this strain of rice.

21. The level of blood sugar varies considerably from individual to individual, day to day, and hour to hour, and on a population level, it displays continuous variation. However, the diagnosis of Type 2 diabetes is set by relatively fixed criteria. A fasting blood sugar level of 126 mg/dL or higher, repeated on different days, is diagnostic of diabetes. A casual (non-fasting) blood sugar level of 200 mg/dL or higher is suggestive of diabetes. In either case, although the level of blood sugar is influenced by a variety of factors (polygenic and environmental), the actual diagnosis of the disease leads one to be classified as diabetic or not diabetic. Because there are only two phenotypic classes (or three if one included the prediabetic state), diabetes is referred to as a threshold trait.

Thus, even though the disease is considered to be polygenic, with multiple genes contributing in an additive fashion, a particular number of additive alleles might be necessary for the trait to be expressed at a detectable or clinical level, and once expressed, additional alleles do not alter the diagnosis. A number of developmental conditions are determined by threshold effects in this way. Interestingly, the threshold may be influenced by gender and/or environmental factors. Because of such complexities, it is often difficult to determine the genetic basis of some human conditions.

Chapter 21: Population and Evolutionary Genetics

Concept Areas	Corresponding Problems
Variation	1, 5, 15, 18, 25, 28
Sequence Analysis	1, 3, 4, 5, 29, 30, 31
Hardy–Weinberg Computations	6, 8, 9, 10, 11, 13, 19, 21, 27
Hardy–Weinberg Assumptions	7, 9, 14, 27, 28
Speciation	1, 2, 4, 15, 23, 25, 26
Mutation	2, 3, 15, 16, 17, 28, 30
Gene Therapy	24
Selection	1, 2, 11, 12, 15, 20
Migration	2, 15, 22
Fitness	10, 20
Inbreeding	13, 19, 21, 27, 29
Evolution	1, 4, 17, 24, 31
Genetic Drift	15, 27, 29

Structures and Processes Checklist–Significant items that deserve special attention are identified with a "*".

(Check topic when mastered–provide examples where appropriate–understand the context of each entry)

- **Overview**
  - evolutionary aspects*
  - neo-Darwinism
  - speciation*
  - environmental diversity
  - microevolution
  - macroevolution
- **Genetic Variation Is Present***
  - population*
  - gene pool*
  - artificial selection*
  - alcohol dehydrogenase (*Adh*) gene
  - nucleotide sequence variation

- next-generation sequencing (NGS)
- genetic variants
- neutral theory
- natural selection
- **The Hardy-Weinberg Law***
  - allele frequencies*
  - genotype frequencies*
  - Hardy-Weinberg law*
  - ideal population
  - $p + q = 1$
  - $p^2 + 2pq + q^2 = 1$
  - no selection*
  - no mutation*

- no migration*
- infinitely large population*
- random mating*
- genetic variability
- **H-W in Human Populations***
  - testing for H-W equilibrium*
  - multiple alleles*
  - $p + q + r = 1$
  - $p^2 + q^2 + r^2 + 2pq + 2pr + 2qr = 1$
- **Natural Selection Drives Change**
  - natural selection*
  - phenotypic variation*
  - variations are heritable*
  - exponential reproduction*
  - competition*
  - successful phenotypes*
  - differential survival and reproduction
  - evolutionary change*
  - detecting natural selection*
  - fitness (w)*
  - decline in frequencies
  - $q_g = \dfrac{q_0}{1 + gq_0}$
  - directional selection*
  - stabilizing selection*
  - disruptive selection*
  - effects on phenotypic mean and variance

- **New Alleles***
  - mutation
  - mutation rate (μ)*
  - indirect methods used for recessive mutations
  - direct measurements used for dominant mutations
  - conditions for direct measurement
  - achondroplasia
- **Migration and Gene Flow***
  - migration*
  - $p_i' = (1 - m)\, p_i + mp_m$
- **Genetic Drift and Small Populations***
  - genetic drift
  - founder effect*
  - genetic bottleneck*
- **Nonrandom Mating***
  - positive assortative mating*
  - negative assortative mating*
  - inbreeding*
  - coefficient of inbreeding (F)*
  - $F = \dfrac{H_e - H_o}{H_e}$
  - consanguineous marriage
- **Reproductive Isolation***
  - species*
  - anagenesis
  - cladogenesis
  - genetic divergence*

- reproductive isolating mechanisms*
- prezygotic isolating mechanisms*
- postzygotic isolating mechanisms*
- speciation*
- geographic barriers
- rate of macroevolution*
- **Evolutionary History***
  - phylogenetic trees*
  - branch
  - node
- tip
- root, or common ancestor
- DNA sequence comparisons
- molecular clocks*
- calibration
- paleogenomics*
- human evolution*
- Denisovans
- Neanderthals*

F21.1 Simple illustration of the relationships among populations, individuals, alleles, and allelic frequencies (p and q).

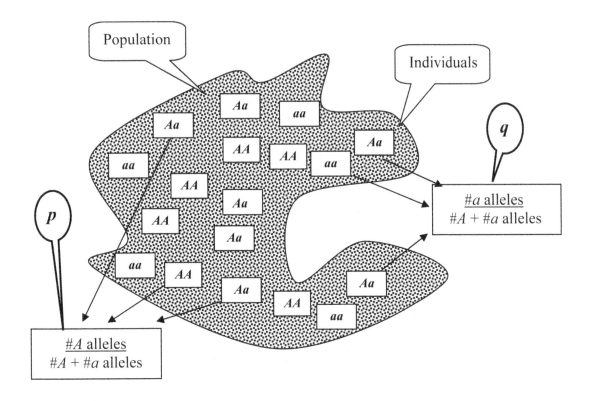

F21.2 Diagram of the relationships among inbreeding, heterozygosity, and homozygosity. Note that as inbreeding occurs, heterozygosity decreases and homozygosity increases.

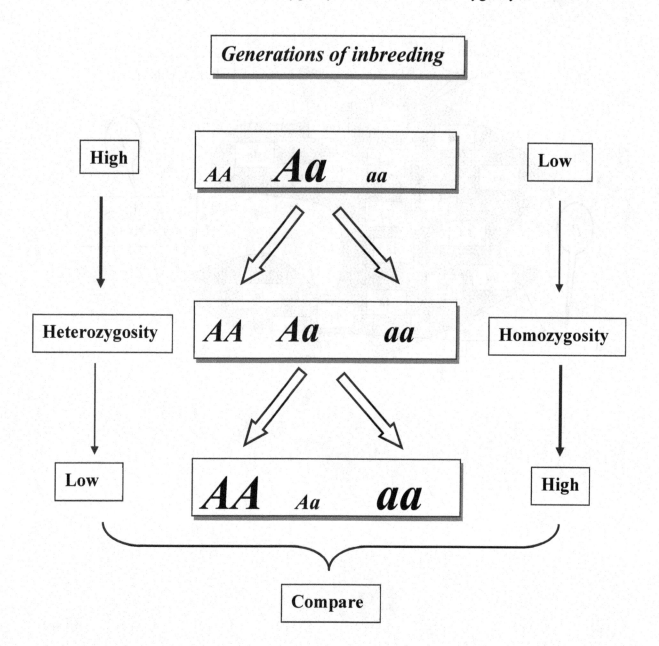

Answers to Now Solve This

21.1 Because the alleles follow a dominant/recessive mode, one can use the formula $\sqrt{q^2}$ to calculate q, on which all other aspects of the answer depend. The frequency of *aa* types is determined by dividing the number of nontasters (37) by the total number of individuals (125).

$q^2 = 37/125 = 0.296$
$q = 0.544$
$p = 1 - q$
$p = 0.456$

The frequencies of the genotypes are determined by applying the formula $p^2 + 2pq + q^2 = 1$ as follows:

Frequency of *AA* $= p^2$
                    $= (0.456)^2$
                    $= 0.208$ or 20.8%

Frequency of *Aa* $= 2pq$
                    $= 2(0.456)(0.544)$
                    $= 0.496$ or 49.6%

Frequency of *aa* $= q^2$
                    $= (0.544)^2$
                    $= 0.296$ or 29.6%

When completing such a set of calculations, it is a good practice to add the final percentages to be certain that they total 100 percent. (Note that this calculation requires the assumption that this population is in Hardy–Weinberg equilibrium with respect to the gene for PTC tasting.)

21.2 (a) For the CCR5 analysis, first determine p and q. You know the frequencies of all the genotypes; therefore, you can calculate p as the sum of 0.6 and $(0.351/2) = 0.7755$; q will be the sum of 0.049, and $(0.351/2) = 0.2245$.

The equilibrium values will be as follows:

Frequency of *1/1* $= p^2 = (0.7755)^2 = 0.6014$ or 60.14%

Frequency of *1/Δ32* $= 2pq = 2(0.7755)(0.2245) = 0.3482$ or 34.82%

Frequency of *Δ32/Δ32* $= q^2 = (0.2245)^2 = 0.0504$ or 5.04%

Comparing these equilibrium values with the observed values strongly suggests that the observed values are drawn from a population in Hardy–Weinberg equilibrium.

(b) For the sickle-cell analysis, first determine p and q. Since the frequencies of all the genotypes are known, one can calculate p as the sum of 0.756 and $(0.242/2) = 0.877$; q will be $(1 - 0.877)$ or 0.123. [NOTE: You can also calculate q as the sum of 0.002 and $(0.242/2) = 0.123$.]

The equilibrium values will be as follows:

Frequency of *SS* $= p^2 = (0.877)^2 = 0.7691$ or 76.91%

Frequency of *Ss* $= 2pq = 2(0.877)(0.123) = 0.2157$ or 21.57%

Frequency of *ss* $= q^2 = (0.123)^2 = 0.0151$ or 1.51%

Comparing these equilibrium values with the observed values suggests that the observed values may be drawn from a population that is not in equilibrium. Notice that there are more heterozygotes than predicted, and fewer homozygotes (especially the *ss* types) than predicted in the population. Because data are given in percentages, χ^2 values cannot be computed.

Chapter 21 Population and Evolutionary Genetics

21.3 The recessive allele a is present in the homozygous state (q^2) at a frequency of 0.0001.

(a) $q = 0.01$

(b) $p = 1 - q$ or 0.99

(c) $2pq = 2(0.01)(0.99) = 0.0198$ (or about 1/50)

(d) $2pq \times 2pq = 0.0198 \times 0.0198 = 0.000392$ (or about 1/2550)

21.4 First, determine the frequency of the CF allele in the general population. Since 1/2500 are affected (q^2), then $q = 1/50$. The frequency of the normal allele is given by $p = 49/50$.

The probability that the woman (with no family history of CF) is heterozygous is $2pq$, or $2(1/50)(49/50)$.

The probability that the man is heterozygous is 2/3.

The probability that a child with CF will be produced by two heterozygotes is 1/4.

Therefore, the overall probability of the couple producing a CF child is $98/2500 \times 2/3 \times 1/4 = 0.00653$, or about 1/153.

Solutions to Problems and Discussion Questions

1. (a) Genetic variation can be assessed in a variety of ways, including responses to artificial selection and sequencing of nucleic acids and proteins.

(b) Different alleles will show typical segregation patterns and have similarities in nucleotide and amino acid sequences.

(c) By conducting assays of gene and/or genotypic frequencies over time and space, one can determine whether the genetic structure of a population is changing.

(d) If gene flow between populations becomes sufficiently reduced, divergence may have reached a point where the populations are reproductively isolated. Under this condition, they are usually considered different species.

(e) Various molecular clocks can be used to estimate the time of divergence of two groups of organisms. Such clocks are based on amino acid and/or nucleotide differences and are often validated by comparison with the fossil record.

2. Your essay should explain how migration (especially when the immigrants have different gene frequencies compared to the host population) and mutation can cause gene frequencies to change in a population. You should also describe selection as resulting from the biased passage of gametes to the next generation. Be sure to include a discussion of the mechanisms of reproductive isolation.

3. (a) Missense mutations cause amino acid changes.

(b) Horizontal transfer refers to the process of passing genetic information from one organism to another without producing offspring. In bacteria, plasmid transfer is an example of horizontal transfer.

(c) The fact that none of the isolates shared identical nucleotide changes indicates that there is little genetic exchange among different strains. Each alteration is unique, most likely originating in an ancestral strain and maintained in descendants of that strain only.

4. The classification of organisms into different species is based on evidence (morphological, genetic, ecological, etc.) that they are reproductively isolated. That is, there must be evidence that gene flow does not occur among the groups being called different species. Classifications above the species level (genus, family, etc.) are not based on such empirical data and are somewhat arbitrary, based on traditions that extend far beyond DNA sequence information. In addition, recall that DNA sequence divergence is not always directly proportional to morphological, behavioral, or ecological divergence. Although the genus classifications provided in this problem seem to be invalid, other factors, beyond simple DNA sequence comparison, must be considered in classification practices. As more information is gained on the meaning of DNA sequence differences in comparison to morphological factors, many phylogenetic relationships will likely be reconsidered, and it is possible that adjustments will be needed in some classification schemes.

5. Many regions of DNA in a eukaryotic genome are not reflected in a protein product. Indeed, many are not even transcribed and/or have no apparent physiological role. Such regions are more likely to tolerate nucleotide changes compared with those that have a necessary physiological impact. Introns, for example, show sequence variation that is not reflected in a protein product. Exons, on the other hand, code for products that are usually involved in production of a phenotype and, as such, are subject to selection.

6. For each of these values, take the square root to determine q, then compute p. Using these values, calculate $2pq$ to determine the number of heterozygotes.

(a) $q = 0.08$; $2pq = 2(0.92)(0.08)$
$\qquad\qquad\qquad = 0.1472$ or 14.72%

(b) $q = 0.009$; $2pq = 2(0.991)(0.009)$
$\qquad\qquad\qquad\quad = 0.01784$ or 1.78%

(c) $q = 0.3$; $2pq = 2(0.7)(0.3)$
$\qquad\qquad\quad = 0.42$ or 42%

(d) $q = 0.1$; $2pq = 2(0.9)(0.1)$
$\qquad\qquad\quad = 0.18$ or 18%

(e) $q = 0.316$; $2pq = 2(0.684)(0.316)$
$\qquad\qquad\qquad\quad = 0.4323$ or 43.23%

(Depending how one rounds off the decimals, slightly different answers will occur.)

7. In order for the Hardy-Weinberg equation to apply, the population must be in Hardy-Weinberg equilibrium.

8. Assuming that the population is in Hardy-Weinberg equilibrium, given the frequency of individuals with the dominant phenotype, the remainder will have the recessive phenotype (q^2). Use this to calculate q and then p. Apply the formula $2pq$ to determine the number of carriers.

9. Given that $q^2 = 0.04$, then $q = 0.2$, $2pq = 0.32$, and $p^2 = 0.64$. Of those individuals *not* expressing the trait, only a mating between heterozygotes can

produce offspring that express the trait, and then only at a frequency of 1/4.

$$Aa \times Aa = 0.32 \times 0.32 = 0.1024$$

Matings between heterozygotes occur about 10 percent of the time. Therefore, one would arrive at a final likelihood of $1/4 \times 10$ percent or 2.5 percent of the offspring having the trait.

10. To calculate the new frequency of the a allele, you need to determine the relative contributions from both surviving aa homozygotes and surviving Aa heterozygotes, each expressed as a proportion of the overall allele contribution of the total surviving population. Thus, the contribution from surviving aa homozygotes would be given as

$$\frac{w_{aa}q^2}{w_{AA}p^2 + w_{Aa}2pq + w_{aa}q^2}$$

and that from surviving Aa heterozygotes given as

$$\frac{w_{Aa}\,pq}{w_{AA}p^2 + w_{Aa}2pq + w_{aa}q^2}$$

The sum of these values will give the frequency of the a allele in the next generation:

$$q_{g+1} = [w_{Aa}p_gq_g + w_{aa}q_g^2]/[w_{AA}p_g^2 + w_{Aa}2p_gq_g + w_{aa}q_g^2]$$

where q_{g+1} is the frequency of the a allele in the next generation, q_g is the frequency of the a allele in this generation, p_g is the frequency of the A allele in this generation, and each "w" represents the fitness of its respective genotype.

(a) $q_{g+1} = [0.9(0.7)(0.3) + 0.8(0.3)^2]/[1(0.7)^2 + 0.9(2)(0.7)(0.3) + 0.8(.3)^2]$

$\qquad q_{g+1} = 0.278$ $\quad p_{g+1} = 0.722$

(b) $q_{g+1} = 0.289$ $\quad p_{g+1} = 0.711$

(c) $q_{g+1} = 0.298$ $\quad p_{g+1} = 0.702$

(d) $q_{g+1} = 0.319$ $\quad p_{g+1} = 0.681$

11. The general equation for responding to this question is

$$q_n = q_0 / (1 + nq_0)$$

where n = the number of generations, q_0 = the initial gene frequency, and q_n = the new gene frequency.

$n = 1$
$\qquad q_1 = 0.5/[1 + (1 \times 0.5)]$
$\qquad q_1 = 0.33$ $\qquad p_1 = 0.67$

n = 5

$q_5 = 0.5/[1 + (5 \times 0.5)]$
$q_5 = 0.143$ $\qquad p_5 = 0.857$

n = 10

$q_{10} = 0.5/[1 + (10 \times 0.5)]$
$q_{10} = 0.083$ $\qquad p_{10} = 0.917$

n = 25

$q_{25} = 0.5/[1 + (25 \times 0.5)]$
$q_{25} = 0.037$ $\qquad p_{25} = 0.963$

n = 100

$q_{100} = 0.5/[1 + (100 \times 0.5)]$
$q_{100} = 0.0098$ $\qquad p_{100} = 0.9902$

n = 1000

$q_{1000} = 0.5/[1 + (1000 \times 0.5)]$
$q_{1000} = 0.000998$ $\quad p_{1000} = 0.999002$

12. Selection against a dominant lethal allele is high, so it is unlikely that it will be present at a high frequency, if at all. However, if the allele shows incomplete penetrance or late age of onset (after reproductive age), it may remain in a population.

13. To solve this problem, predict the probability of one of the grandparents being heterozygous.

Given the frequency of the disorder in the population as 1 in 10,000 individuals (0.0001), then $q^2 = 0.0001$, and $q = 0.01$. The frequency of heterozygosity is $2pq$, or approximately 0.02, as also stated in the problem. The probability for one *or* the other of the grandparents to be heterozygous would therefore be the sum of the individual probabilities, or 0.02 + 0.02, which is 0.04 or 1/25.

If one of the grandparents is a carrier, then the probability of the offspring from a first-cousin mating being homozygous for the recessive gene is 1/64. Multiplying the two probabilities together gives $1/64 \times 1/25 = 1/1600$. (Note: If one considers the probability of both grandparents being carriers, 0.02×0.02, the answer differs slightly.)

The population at large has a frequency of homozygous recessive individuals of 1/10,000; therefore, one can easily see how inbreeding increases the likelihood of homozygosity.

14. The frequency of an allele is determined by a number of factors, including the fitness it confers, mutation rate, and input from migration. The distribution of a gene among individuals is determined by mating (population size, inbreeding, etc.) and environmental factors (selection, etc.). If a population is in Hardy-Weinberg equilibrium, the distribution of genotypes occurs at or around the $p^2 + 2pq + q^2 = 1$ expression (see F21.1). Equilibrium does not mean 25 percent *AA*, 50 percent *Aa*, and 25 percent *aa*. This confusion often stems from the 1:2:1 (or 3:1) ratio seen in Mendelian crosses.

15. During speciation, individuals or groups of potentially interbreeding organisms become genetically distinct from other members of the species. Members of different populations with substantial genetic divergence are, at first, not reproductively isolated from each other, although gene flow might be restricted. The distinction between such groups is not absolute in that one group might attempt mating with other groups of the species. Any process that favors changes in allele frequencies has the potential of generating substantial genetic differences among different populations.

Factors such as selection, migration, genetic drift, or even mutation might be important in generating significant genetic change. One would certainly include geographic isolation as a major barrier to gene flow and thus an important process in such formation.

Natural selection occurs when there is nonrandom elimination of individuals from a population. Because such selection is a strong force in changing allele frequencies, it should also be considered as a significant factor in subspecies formation.

16. Three of the affected infants had affected parents —the most likely explanation for their mutations is inheritance of an existing mutation. Therefore, only two "new" mutations enter into the problem. The allele is dominant, so each new case of achondroplasia arose from a single new mutation. There are 50,000 births (and 100,000 gametes). The frequency of mutation is, therefore, given as follows: 2/100,000 or 2×10^{-5}.

17. The approximate similarity of mutation rates among genes and lineages should provide more credible estimates of divergence times of species and allow for broader interpretations of sequence comparisons. It also provides for increased understanding of the mutational processes that govern evolution among mammalian genomes. For example, if the rate of mutation is fairly constant among lineages or cells that have a more rapid turnover, it indicates that replication-related errors do not make a significant contribution to mutation rates.

18. The presence of selectively neutral alleles and genetic adaptations to varied environments contribute significantly to genetic variation in natural populations.

19. Since $r1 = 0.81$ and $r2 = 0.19$, the expected frequency of heterozygotes would be $2pq \times 125$ or $2(0.81 \times 0.19) \times 125 = 38.475$. The observed frequency is 20. The inbreeding coefficient (F) is given by:

$F = (H_e - H_o)/H_e$

$F = (38.475 - 20)/38.475 = 0.48$

20. Given that only 10 percent of the sensitive (bb) corn borer larvae feeding on Bt corn plants survive, fitness, $w_{bb} = 0.1$. Plants with at least one B allele survive; therefore, $w_{BB} = 1$ and $w_{Bb} = 1$. The B allele for resistance exists at an initial frequency of 0.02 (represented as p); therefore, $q = 0.98$. The frequency of the b allele after one generation of corn borers fed on Bt corn would be computed as follows:

$q_{g+1} = [w_{Bb}p_gq_g + w_{bb}q_g^2]/[w_{BB}p_g^2 + w_{Bb}2p_gq_g + w_{bb}q_g^2]$

(See the answer to problem 10 for an explanation of this equation.)

$q_{g+1} = [1(0.02)(0.98) + (0.1)(0.98)^2] /$

$\qquad [1(0.02)^2 + 1(2)(0.02)(0.98) + (0.1)(0.98)^2]$

$q_{g+1} = 0.852$ and $p_{g+1} = 0.148$

21. The following distribution of genotypes occurs among the 50 desert bighorn sheep in which the normal dominant C allele produces straight coats.

$CC = 29$ straight coats

$Cc = 17$ straight coats

$cc = 4$ curled coats

Computing, $p = 0.75$ and $q = 0.25$, which gives $2pq = 0.375$ for the expected frequency of heterozygotes. Since 17/50 or 0.34 are observed as heterozygotes, the coefficient of inbreeding (F) is

$F = (H_e - H_o)/H_e$

$F = (0.375 - 0.34)/0.375 = 0.093$

This problem could also be solved using the actual numbers of sheep in each category, where there would be 18.75 heterozygotes expected $(2pq)(50)$:

$F = (18.75 - 17)/18.75 = 0.093$.

22. The equation for determining the impact of immigration on the gene pool of an existing population is estimated by the following equation:

$$p_i^{'} = (1 - m)\, p_i + mp_m$$

Substituting in the appropriate values produces the following expression:

$p_i^{'} = (1 - 0.167)(0.75) + (0.167)(1.0)$

$p_i^{'} = 0.792$ and $q_i^{'} = 0.208$

Note that the value of 0.167 comes from the fact that 10 sheep are introduced into an existing population of 50, so 10/60 (or 16.7 percent) of the parents of the next generation are migrants. Also note that there are no c alleles in the introduced population, so $p_m = 1.0$.

23. In general, speciation involves the gradual accumulation of genetic changes to a point where reproductive isolation occurs. Depending on environmental or geographic conditions, genetic changes may occur slowly or rapidly. They can involve point mutations or chromosomal changes.

24. Somatic gene therapy, like any therapy, allows some individuals to live more normal lives than those not receiving therapy. As such, the ability of these individuals to contribute to the gene pool increases the likelihood that less fit alleles will enter and be maintained in the gene pool. This is a normal consequence of therapy, genetic or not, and in the face of disease control and prevention, societies have generally accepted this consequence. Germ-line therapy could, if successful, lead to limited, isolated, and infrequent removal of an allele from a gene lineage. However, given the present state of the science, its impact on the course of human evolution will be diluted and negated by a host of other factors that afflict humankind.

25. Reproductive isolating mechanisms include the following:

- Geographic or ecological; same region but different habitats

- Seasonal or temporal; same region but different mating maturation

- Behavioral; incompatible courtship behaviors

- Mechanical; reproductive structures inhibit or restrict mating

- Physiological; gametic nonviability

- Hybrid nonviability or weakness

- Developmental hybrid sterility

- Segregational hybrid sterility

- F_2 breakdown, progeny of hybrids have reduced fertility

26. Reproductive isolating mechanisms are grouped into prezygotic and postzygotic. Prezygotic mechanisms are more efficient because they occur before resources are expended in the processes of mating.

27. (a) The gene is most likely autosomal because there is no indication that males are disproportionally affected. It is recessive because all affected individuals have unaffected parents. For the population, $q^2 = 0.002$, so $q = 0.045$, $p = 0.955$, and $2(pq) = 0.086$.

(b) The "founder effect" is probably operating here. Relatively small, local populations that are relatively isolated in a reproductive sense tend to show differences in gene frequencies when compared with larger populations. In such small populations, homozygosity is increased as a gene has a higher probability of "meeting itself."

28. In small populations, large fluctuations in gene frequency occur because random gametic sampling may not include all the genetic variation in the parents. The same phenomenon occurs in molecular populations. Two factors can cause the extinction of a particular mutation in small populations. First, sampling error may allow fixation of one form and the elimination of others. If an advantageous mutation occurs, it must be included in the next replicative round in order to be maintained in subsequent generations. If the founding population is small, it is possible that the advantageous mutation might not be represented. Second, although the previous statements also hold for deleterious mutations, if a deleterious mutation becomes fixed, it can lead to extinction of that population.

29. When a population bottleneck occurs and the number of effective breeders is reduced, two phenomena usually follow. First, because the population is small, wide fluctuations in genotypic frequencies occur, thereby revealing deleterious alleles by chance. Second, inbreeding often occurs in small populations, thereby increasing the chance for homozygosity. With increased homozygosity comes an increased likelihood that recessive alleles will be expressed. Because many disease-causing genes are recessive, an increase in genetic diseases is a likely aftermath to a population bottleneck.

30. With one exception (the final amino acid in the sequences), all of the amino acid substitutions (Ala to Gly, Val to Leu, Asp to Asn, and Met to Leu) require only one nucleotide change. The last change, Pro (CCN) to Lys (AAA, G), requires two changes (the minimal mutational distance).

31. In general, calibrating molecular data such as amino acid and nucleotide substitutions to absolute times of divergence is usually done by comparison with the existing fossil record. This method is, however, subject to error due to uncertainty of the fossil record and because different mutation rates, generation times, and population structures occur among different taxa.

Review and Discussion Questions (Special Topics #1): Epigenetics

Review Question Answers

1. The major epigenetic alterations of the genome include DNA methylation; reversible histone modification (acetylation, methylation, and phosphorylation); chromatin remodeling; binding of microRNAs; and long noncoding RNAs. It is likely that additional epigenetic mechanisms await discovery.

2. In mammals, methylation of cytosine residues, when it occurs, takes place at CpG-rich regions in promoters and upstream sequences. The effect is to block transcription, thereby silencing the genes. The majority of methylated sequences in mammals are found in heterochromatin, where they promote chromatin stability by preventing replication and transcription of transposable elements.

3. Several groups of proteins are involved in histone modification. Some proteins (writers) add chemical groups to histones, others interpret modifications (readers), and some remove the added chemical groups (erasers). Such modifications influence the structure of chromatin by altering the accessibility of nucleosomes, and render the chromatin either "open" or "closed" for transcription.

4. Reversible modifications of histone tails alter the ability of histones (and therefore nucleosomes) to bind tightly to DNA. Modifications that weaken this interaction make the chromatin more accessible to interactions with other proteins, such as the transcriptional machinery. Conversely, modifications that strengthen this interaction make the chromatin less accessible.

5. The histone code describes the patterns of reversible posttranslational modifications of histones and the interactions between and among them that contribute to the regulation of gene expression.

6. Imprinting usually involves specific genes that are restricted in number and that are altered by passage through meiosis. Whereas most genomic methylation patterns are reversed at fertilization, imprinting is not. A gene that is marked by a maternally derived imprint will not have a paternally derived imprint and vice versa. Imprinted sequences are the same in all cells of an organism and, in somatic cells, are permanent. Imprinted alleles are transcriptionally silent in all cells. Epigenetic modifications (methylation, histone modification, interaction with ncRNAs), by contrast, are generally reversible and can be responsive to environmental signals.

7. Changes in nucleosome spacing is directly correlated with changes in gene expression. DNA methylation and histone alterations work in concert to regulate access of proteins to DNA. When DNA is unmethylated and histones are acetylated, nucleosomes are spaced apart—in the open configuration—making DNA more accessible and allowing transcription to occur. When DNA is methylated and histones are deacetylated, nucleosomes are relatively close together—in the closed configuration. In this circumstance, DNA is inaccessible and transcription is suppressed.

8. Most imprinted genes are found clustered on chromosomes and generally encode growth factors or genes that regulate such factors. Mutations in the imprinting of genes (epimutations) are caused either by changes in DNA sequence or by dysfunctional epigenetic changes. Both can result in heritable changes in gene activity. Dysfunctional imprinting is especially dangerous, since changes in methylation for one imprinted gene often affect the expression of adjacent or coordinately controlled imprinted genes within a cluster. Imprinted genes generally act early in development, so defects in their expression have serious consequences. Some diseases caused by faulty imprinting include Prader–Willi syndrome, Angelman syndrome, and Beckwith–Wiedemann syndrome.

Discussion Question Answers

1. There is evidence both in mice and in humans that epigenetic disorders might be treatable *in utero*, at least on a limited scale. In mice, coat color under the control of the metastable epiallele A^{vy} ranges from pseudoagouti to fully yellow, depending on the methylation status of a promoter element. Pregnant female mice whose diet included methylation precursors gave birth to offspring whose coat color was less varied and more resembled pseudoagouti (the more methylated phenotype). In humans, demethylation treatments have been applied to human disorders [such as Vidaza (azacytidine), a

DNA methyltransferase inhibitor used to treat cancer]. However, because DNA methylation is a common and significant component of normal genetic regulation, what may be useful for controlling one gene in the genome may cause numerous unwanted changes in other parts of the genome.

2. Studies show there is a four- to nine-fold increased risk of a child conceived via ART having Beckwith–Wiedemann syndrome. Increased incidences of Prader–Willi syndrome and Angelman syndrome have also been reported. Children conceived by IVF who have one of these syndromes have reduced levels or loss of maternal-specific imprinting. Furthermore, the time frame of ART manipulations coincides with the timing of epigenetic reprogramming, giving weight to the hypothesis that the manipulation of embryos interferes with imprinting. Given these data, it would seem reasonable that such information should be provided to prospective ART users. Each couple would need to reach a decision based on available science and their own value and belief sets.

3. Mutations in tumor-suppressor genes and proto-oncogenes (or their regulatory elements) are necessary components for cancer formation, but they are not sufficient. Other factors, including additional mutations or lack of DNA repair, are also needed for a cell to become malignant. Epigenetic changes are known to modify gene expression and could have a role in development of cancer. For example, loss of heterozygosity could be explained by hypermethylation of the promoter of the otherwise undamaged allele.

4. Some RNAs (such as miRNAs and lncRNAs) are known to downregulate gene expression. According to the study, some foods could be the source of regulatory RNAs that circulate in body fluids of humans. Further studies would need to show from which plants the regulatory RNAs are derived, which genes are affected, and at what levels these RNAs are required to significantly alter gene expression before informed decisions can be made regarding safety. At this point it might be premature to design a dietary regimen based on such a frail understanding of the role of plant RNAs in humans.

Review and Discussion Questions (Special Topics #2): Genetic Testing

Review Question Answers

1. A diagnostic test seeks to identify a mutation or change that causes a disease. Some examples of diagnostic tests are the use of amniocentesis followed by karyotype analysis to identify trisomies, or the use of ASOs to determine whether an individual is a carrier of the sickle-cell allele. Prognostic testing, by contrast, is done to determine the likelihood that a person will develop a particular disease. One example of this is the use of GWAS to identify SNPs that are associated with the occurrence of a particular disorder, such as Type 2 diabetes. Statistical analysis of the data is required to determine the extent of the risk of developing a disease phenotype.

2. Prognostic tests are predictive whereas diagnostic tests identify mutations. Scenarios (a) and (d) are prognostic (the mutations are "associated with" or "correlated with" the disorders), while scenarios (b), (c), and (e) are diagnostic.

3. In the United States, requirements for newborn screening are determined on a state-by-state basis and not federally. Currently, all states require some form of genetic testing. Although the federal government does not set requirements, the Department of Health and Human Services does recommend testing for 34 specific conditions (see the Recommended Uniform Screening Panel, or RUSP, list).

4. Experimental conditions in an ASO test allow hybridization only when the test and probe sequences show 100 percent complementarity (a perfect match). Alleles that differ by even a single nucleotide can be distinguished. In this case, DNA from an individual that is homozygous recessive for the sickle-cell allele will hybridize strongly to the probe for the mutant allele (the β^S probe) but not to the wild-type probe (the β^A probe).

5. ASOs are short oligonucleotides that hybridize to their complementary strands in the genome. Since methylation does not interfere with base pairing, an ASO test would be unable to identify epigenetic DNA modifications.

6. Preimplantation genetic diagnosis is used to screen the genomes of embryos created by *in vitro* fertilization for chromosomal abnormalities or for a specific genetic defect, to determine which of the IVF embryos will be introduced into the uterus for implantation.

7. It is possible to isolate DNA and RNA from the same cells, allowing analysis of both the genome and transcriptome simultaneously. DNA can be sequenced and gene expression can be determined using DNA microarrays or by RNA sequencing (and single-cell RNA sequencing). This is important to the diagnosis and treatment of diseases because it accounts for the heterogeneity of target cells in diseases such as cancer. Knowing this, the targeting of treatment can be improved.

8. Microarrays can be used as platforms on which to hybridize DNA or RNA from various tissues. RNA populations from different tissues will give different patterns of hybridization, a so-called transcriptome analysis, identifying which genes are expressed and at what level.

9. Simple sequencing has led to the development of new technologies, such as whole-genome and whole-exome sequencing, as well as genome-wide association studies. These technologies allow for the discovery of mutations that might be associated with certain diseases. Personal genomics, in which individual genomes are sequenced, allow for screening of individuals to help assess their risk of developing a disease or the potential efficacy of a treatment plan. Microarrays can be used to monitor RNA expression levels of thousands of genes in virtually any cell population. By comparing patterns in normal and diseased tissues, scientists can determine which genes are active or inactive under various circumstances. Furthermore, single-cell techniques allow the simultaneous analysis of the genome and the transcriptome. Use of these techniques can, therefore, lead to more precise diagnosis, determination of the efficacy of particular therapies, and refinement of possible therapies.

10. Genome-wide association studies involve scanning the genomes of thousands of unrelated individuals with a particular disease and comparing them with the genomes of individuals who do not have the disease. GWAS attempt to identify genes and mutations that influence disease risk and to make substantial contributions to the diagnosis and treatment of genetic diseases.

11. The term "incidental results" refers to the discovery of additional disease markers or mutations during an analysis of genetic testing results that were gathered to address a particular gene locus or disorder.

Discussion Question Answers

1. Full medical histories from the woman, including previous surgeries (such as the transplant surgeries mentioned), stem cell treatments, previous pregnancies, and recent blood transfusions would prove helpful.

2. Since both mutations occur in the CF gene, children who possess both mutant alleles will develop CF—neither allele will be able to produce a wild-type CF protein. Because both parents are heterozygotes, there is a 25-percent probability that any child will inherit both mutant alleles and develop CF.

3. At this point, there is, understandably, considerable reluctance to allow the open sharing of genetic information among institutions. In general, the establishment of governmental databases containing our most intimate information is viewed with skepticism. It is likely that considerable time and discussion will elapse before such databases are established.

4. Widespread screening of newborns would allow the identification of a virtually infinite number of variables associated with the human genome that might be of scientific and personal interest. Some new bases for certain disease states might be identified. However, disadvantages would be the likely stigmatizing of certain individuals and numerous issues of privacy invasion and discrimination.

5. A number of ethical problems are evident. The means by which the school administration obtained the information that the boy had a mutation in the *CFTR* gene should be questioned, since he showed no symptoms. In addition, the administration used this private genetic information to discriminate against the boy, dismissing him from the school and depriving him of opportunities (both educational and social) that were freely open to others. Furthermore,

the administration appears to have publicly shared this information, which could lead to discriminatory treatment by others.

6. Positive consequences include increasing awareness of the disease, the genetic test, and possible treatment options. Negative consequences include rash decisions made by individuals based solely on the decision of a highly public persona. Each person must decide how to make use of their own genetic information. What is a sound decision for one individual might not be appropriate for another. Hopefully, those individuals making such life-altering decisions will do so with sound information from the scientific community and sufficient understanding of the ramifications of such decisions.

7. Certainly, information provided to physicians and patients about genetic testing is a strong point in favor of wide distribution. It would probably be helpful for companies involved in genetic testing to participate by providing information specific to their operations. It would be helpful if pooled statistical data were made available to the public in terms of frequencies of false positives and negatives, as well as population and/or geographical distributions. It would be necessary, however, that any individual results from tests be held in strict confidence.

8. FDA regulation is one way to decrease the distribution of misinformation that could be associated with such tests. It would also ensure a standard of practice among all companies that could improve the reliability of the results and increase consumer protection.

9. It is a highly personal decision to have one's genome sequenced. However, doing so might identify variations that could be alarming, but have no consequences. Such "false positives" could have a negative impact on an individual. In addition, one must consider a variety of consequences associated with a publicly available genome sequence: employment bias, insurance bias, effect on personal relationships, and so on.

10. It is likely that investigators were looking for some reason to explain the killer's behavior— possibly SNPs correlated with a particular mental illness or tendency to violence, or perhaps even a specific genetic mutation. Given the present state of understanding of behavioral genetics, however, it is unlikely that any definitive conclusions could be reached by such an analysis.

11. Services currently available from 23andMe include two packages: (1) analysis of ancestry (ancestry composition, haplogroups, Neanderthal ancestry) and (2) ancestry plus health analysis (the features of package 1 plus reports presented for health risk, wellness, carrier status, and physical traits); both packages include access to one's raw data and an option to share data with friends and family. Raw genomic information is difficult to interpret without training, and regulation of such companies, especially when health-related information is provided could be beneficial to protect consumers' interests.

12. Because a gene is a product of the natural world, it does not conform to patentable matter as governed by U.S. patent laws. However, the direct-to-consumer test for the *BRCA1* and *BRCA2* genes is original in its process or development, so it should be patentable.

Review and Discussion Questions (Special Topics #3): Gene Therapy

Review Question Answers

1. Gene therapy involves the placement of potentially beneficial genes into a person's cells in an effort to correct some faulty genetic state.

2. In *ex vivo* gene therapy, a potential genetic correction takes place in cells that have been removed from the patient and are subsequently reintroduced into the patient. *In vivo* gene therapy treats cells of the body through the introduction of DNA into affected cells of the patient.

3. In general, integration of the therapeutic DNA into the host genome is advantageous because the stability of the introduced DNA is enhanced, which provides long-term expression; however, the integration process itself may generate mutations and regulatory alterations. There are some applications in which the introduced DNA is not integrated. In these cases, the introduced DNA is usually less stable and repeated infusions are required.

4. In many cases, therapeutic DNA hitches a ride with genetically engineered viruses, such as retrovirus or adenovirus vectors. Nonviral delivery methods may use chemical assistance to cross cell membranes, nanoparticles, or cell fusion with artificial vesicles.

5. Genetically engineered viruses that carry therapeutic DNA infect patient cells and deliver their payloads. Two types of viruses have been used for gene therapy; nonintegrating viruses, exemplified by adeno-associated virus (AAV) and integrating viruses, exemplified by lentiviruses (a type of retrovirus). AAV delivers its DNA into the nucleus, where it exists as an episome and serves as a template for RNA synthesis under the control of viral promoters. These episomes do not replicate, so if delivery is targeted to replicating cells, multiple infusions are needed. Retroviruses deliver their RNA to the cytoplasm, where it is reverse transcribed. The resulting cDNA is imported into the nucleus, where it integrates and is expressed. There remain significant challenges to overcome if gene therapy is to be a safe and effective treatment. The introduction of some viruses can trigger immune responses in patients, which can render the treatment ineffective. While the use of disabled viruses seems to cause fewer problems, there is the possibility that disabled viruses could recombine with an unmodified virus and regain their full infectivity. If integration is desired, it only occurs in replicating cells and, when it does, can be very problematic. Integration directed by integrase directs insertion to active genes, potentially leading to unexpected interruptions of normal host gene functions. In addition, there are questions of how to regulate the expression of the introduced DNA.

6. White blood cells, T cells in this case, were used because they are key players in the mounting of an immune response, which Ashanti was incapable of developing. A normal copy of the *ADA* gene was engineered into a retroviral vector, which then infected many of her T cells. Those cells that expressed the *ADA* gene were then injected into Ashanti's bloodstream, and some of them populated her bone marrow. At the time of Ashanti's treatment, targeted gene therapy was not possible, so integration of the *ADA* gene into Ashanti's genome probably did not replace her defective gene.

7. There have been successes in treatment of diseases in addition to the treatment of ADA-SCID. Hemophilia B is a blood disorder in which patients cannot produce one of the clotting proteins, factor IX. In an initial trial, an adeno-associated virus vector (AAV8) carrying the factor IX gene was introduced into liver cells. These were injected as a single dose into six adult hemophilia patients, four of whom successfully discontinued infusion treatment.

8. Genome editing involves the removal, correction, or replacement of a defective gene, whereas traditional gene therapy involves the addition of a therapeutic gene that coexists with the defective copy. Genome editing can alter one or several bases of a gene or replace the gene entirely. To some extent, genome editing is designed to alleviate one of the major pitfalls of gene therapy, random DNA integration.

9. One key feature of gene editing by CRISPR-Cas is that it can be performed directly in living, adult animals. Furthermore, sequence-specific targeting is easily achieved, driven by complementary base-pairing between the single-stranded guide RNA and the DNA target. Gene replacement takes advantage of endogenous homologous recombination repair to insert donor template DNA. Finally, although off-target edits have occurred, they are rare and fidelity can be improved by careful construction of the sgRNA. Overall, the technique allows precise and specific edits in an efficient and economical manner.

10. ZFNs, or zinc-finger nucleases, consist of a DNA cutting domain from a restriction endonuclease and a DNA-binding domain containing a zinc-finger motif, which can be engineered to recognize any sequence. The zinc-finger motifs bind to the DNA recognition sequence five to seven nucleotides apart from each other and the nuclease domain cuts the DNA between them. The resulting double-strand break can be repaired by homologous recombination or non-homologous end-joining. Targeted gene therapy is possible when ZFNs are combined with integrases and homologous DNA sequences.

11. RNA interference (RNAi) and the use of antisense RNA are two techniques that have been used to silence gene expression. In RNA interference (RNAi), short double-stranded RNA molecules are delivered into cells and are cleaved (by the enzyme Dicer) into relatively short pieces of RNA (siRNA). These associate with an enzyme complex (RNA-induced silencing complex or RISC), which targets mRNA and either prevents its translation or leads to its degradation. In the second technique, an RNA molecule that is complementary to the target, sense mRNA strand (thus, an antisense RNA molecule) is introduced into cells. The antisense RNA binds to its complementary mRNA strand, thus blocking its translation. In either case, the silencing of deleterious or overactive genes may help alleviate disease symptoms, at least on a temporary basis.

Discussion Question Answers

1. Many human conditions are the result of multiple mutations at multiple gene loci, making them too complicated for currently available treatments. For less complex genetic conditions, selection of a suitable vector that does not create a new set of problems (immune response, poor penetration into cells, etc.), will be necessary for widespread use. One major challenge is the problem of integration of therapeutic genes. For current methods in which this occurs, integration is random but often directed to active genes. The challenge is to target integration, so as not to compromise the normal function of other genes in the genome. In addition, the appropriate regulation of introduced DNA must be achieved before such techniques can become commonplace.

2. Currently, gene therapy is considered to be acceptable for the relief of genetic disease states. Given its expense, however, its use is the subject of considerable debate. It remains to be seen whether insurance companies will embrace what might be considered experimental treatments. Use of gene therapy to enhance the competitive status of individuals (genetic enhancement or gene doping) is presently viewed as cheating by most organizations and the public. Finally, it is unlikely that germ-line therapy will be viewed favorably by the public or scientific communities; however, this and other issues mentioned here will be the subject of considerable future debate.

3. Health-care cost is a complex and highly emotionally charged issue. The price of most drugs is higher than the cost to produce them, and many people are asking whether this is justifiable. On the one hand, drug companies are businesses with a responsibility to their shareholders to maximize profit. In addition, the companies argue that they need to recover the cost of research and development in addition to the cost of production to be able to continue ongoing drug development. On the other hand, affected individuals often constitute a small market for each of these expensive drugs; consequently, there is no high demand that might help to lower the cost. Many patients with debilitating genetic diseases cannot afford the often life-saving medication and rely on insurance for help. The cost of insurance is, in part, determined by the number of individuals who pay into the company, the amount of money expended by the company, and the amount of money projected to be spent. Insurance companies are also businesses and need to make a profit to remain in operation. Clearly, this complex issue requires cool-headed discussions that involve all parties.

4. Germ-line and embryo therapy is controversial for a number of reasons, primary among them being the fact that any genomic changes made will persist through future generations. In addition, there are concerns about human experimentation in general and experimentation involving embryos, who are unable to give consent, in particular. There are also safety issues to consider, including that the treatment would need to be shown to be effective and efficient. Side effects, specifically effects of mistargeting, would need to be documented, quantified, and addressed. Further, the potential for altered viability of treated germ cells and embryos would also need to be addressed.

5. The widespread use of gene therapy in the future will depend on its success rate, which encompasses the degree to which diseases are treatable, the attending side effects, and the absence of catastrophic failures. Because many approaches are now being studied, ranging from gene editing to gene replacement to antisense therapies to targeted integration, it is likely that one or more approaches will become viable in treating genetic diseases. Incentives are in place to reward such research should treatments break through the practical and scientific barriers that were discussed in the text.

Review and Discussion Questions (Special Topics #4): Advances in Neurogenetics: The Study of Huntington Disease

Review Question Answers

1. Sequence variations among individuals can create or abolish restriction enzyme recognition sites, producing different lengths of fragments upon digestion with a given restriction enzyme. These variations in fragment sizes are called restriction fragment length polymorphisms or RFLPs. RFLP markers are sometimes linked to disease loci, such that a particular pattern, or haplotype, is associated with the inheritance of the disease allele. James Gusella showed linkage between inheritance of the C haplotype of the G8 RFLP marker and inheritance of the HD locus. When the G8 marker was used in a Southern blot analysis to probe DNA from human–mouse somatic hybrid cells, hybridization was detected only in DNA from hybrid cells carrying human chromosome 4.

2. Not only did Nancy Wexler and her team gather extensive pedigree information, they also collected blood samples from some individuals in each pedigree. DNA isolated from these samples was used to determine genotypes for the donors, allowing James Gusella to establish that the HD locus and the C haplotype of the G8 RFLP marker are coinherited.

3. The mutant protein (mHTT) contains an extended region of polyglutamine residues, which causes protein misfolding. Misfolded proteins subsequently clump together to form aggregates.

4. The results of experiments using an inducible system showed that protein aggregation in the brain and the resulting motor symptoms could be reversed when the mutant *HTT* gene was silenced shortly after the appearance of motor symptoms. This suggested that the disease might be controlled or reversed if treated during the early stages.

5. Mouse models indicated that the whole HTT protein is not needed. The presence of the first exon (which contains the CAG repeat region) has been shown to be sufficient to cause the abnormalities seen in HD.

6. Early mouse models showed that the presence of the promoter and a copy of the first exon, which contained expanded CAG repeats, caused protein aggregation and abnormal neurotransmitter levels, similar to the pathology seen in human brains with HD. As stated in the answer to question 5, the presence of the CAG repeat region seems to be necessary and sufficient for disease manifestation.

7. Binding of mHTT to the outer mitochondrial membrane inhibits the electron transport chain, lowering the amount of available ATP and increasing the levels of reactive oxygen species, which cause cellular damage. Mutant HTT also reduces the numbers of mitochondria. The reduction in ATP production leads to the inability to produce sufficient energy to support cellular functions and the triggering of apoptosis.

8. The use of stem cells is a promising treatment strategy that has recently been tested in mice. Transgenic mice carrying a full-length copy of the human *HTT* gene (*HTT* mice) were injected with human stem cells that were engineered to overexpress brain-derived neurotrophic factor, a required protein for striatal brain cells. A significant decrease in the HD phenotype, longer lifespan, and increased nerve cell production were observed.

Gene silencing is another strategy to reduce levels of mHTT. Two strategies were tested in mice. (1) Repression of m*HTT* transcription by gene editing using ZFNs: The ZFN constructs (initially tested in mouse and human culture cells) were delivered into *HTT* mice by injection into the striatal region of one side of the brain. A reduction of m*HTT* mRNA was observed on the injected side. (2) Degradation of target mRNA using complementary ASOs: ASOs were delivered to *HTT* mice by transfusion into the cerebrospinal fluid. Levels of the mutant mRNA and protein were reduced and HD symptoms improved. Phase I clinical trials in humans began in 2015.

Genome editing using CRISPR-Cas9: Separate constructs for Cas9 and for sgRNAs specific for the m*HTT* gene were injected into the striatum of transgenic mice carrying exon 1 of the human m*HTT* gene. Results indicated decreased mHTT levels, reduced protein aggregation, and improved motor skills.

Discussion Question Answers

1. The polyglutamine sequences encoded by mutant genes with expanded CAG repeat regions not only cause misfolding and aggregation, but (in the case of mHTT) also allow the mutant proteins to participate in interactions in which the normal proteins do not. These include transcriptional repression, inhibition of chaperones, and induction of apoptosis, among others. It makes sense that these nine neurodegenerative diseases share a common mechanism, since they share the same general defect.

2. Prioritizing understanding of the functions and mechanisms of the mutant HTT protein is necessary for the development and assessment of treatment strategies. However, it is critical for any potential treatment to specifically target the mutant protein and not also inhibit the normal protein. Therefore, understanding of the function and mechanisms of the *normal* HTT protein is equally important.

3. The use of stem cell transplants to replace damaged cells might slow progression of the disease and help to alleviate some symptoms. However, if these healthy cells can take up mutant HTT, they will eventually succumb, and the benefits of treatment will be only temporary. Therefore, stem cell therapy would not be effective.

4. As we learned in Chapter 4 and revisited in Chapter 6, trinucleotide repeat diseases (such as myotonic dystrophy, fragile-X syndrome, or HD) show genetic anticipation, in which the disease appears earlier and with greater severity in each successive generation. Anticipation has been correlated with increases in the number of repeats in each case.

5. There are many ethical issues to consider. The most obvious center around privacy and the potential for discrimination—especially by employers or life and health insurance providers. But there are also more subtle ethical issues. For example, the question of whether adults with the m*HTT* allele should be allowed to give consent to have their children tested or to have prenatal tests performed on embryos or fetuses. Some other questions are: What should be the obligations of physicians to provide counseling, both genetic and psychological, to a patient whose parent has HD? Should a physician urge an at-risk patient to undergo diagnostic testing? Should patients who have the m*HTT* allele be required to seek genetic counseling before conceiving a child?

Review and Discussion Questions (Special Topics #5): DNA Forensics

Review Question Answers

1. VNTR profiling is a form of DNA profiling that takes advantage of the variable number of tandem repeats (VNTRs) that are located in various regions of the genome. Such repeats are generally made up of DNA sequences between 15 and 100 bp in length. Their use in DNA profiling rests in the fact that the number of repeats varies from person to person and there are multiple alleles (up to 30) for each locus. VNTRs can be used to match a DNA sample recovered from a given circumstance (crime, organismic remains, paternity testing, ancient lineage, etc.) with other DNA samples.

2. STRs are like VNTRs, but the repeat portion is shorter, between two and nine base pairs, repeated from 7 to 40 times. With the development of the polymerase chain reaction, even trace amounts of DNA samples can be analyzed relatively quickly. A core set of STR loci (20 in the United States and 12 in Europe) is most often used in forensic applications.

3. Capillary electrophoresis uses thin glass tubes containing polyacrylamide gel onto which fluorescently labeled amplified DNA is loaded. Electrophoresis separates the DNA fragments by size and detects each labeled fragment. From the resulting electropherogram, the amount and length of each fragment can be determined. Although the original template DNA is present in amplified samples, it is unlabeled and will be "invisible" to the fluorescence detectors.

4. Males typically contain a Y chromosome and females do not (exceptions include transgender and mosaic individuals); therefore, gender identification as well as gender separation in a mixed tissue sample is easily achieved by Y chromosome profiling. In addition, STR profiling is possible for more than 200 loci; however, because of the relative stability of DNA in the Y chromosome, it is difficult to differentiate DNA from fathers and sons, male siblings or any male from the same patrilineage.

5. SNP profiling uses single-nucleotide polymorphisms (SNPs) that occur randomly at millions of loci in the human genome, whereas STR profiling uses repeated sequences of 2–9 nucleotides in length. Both techniques amplify target regions of the sample by PCR prior to analysis. While STR profiling detects alleles by the different sizes of the amplified products, SNP alleles are detected by hybridization to allele-specific probes or by sequence analysis. Because only small segments of DNA are required for SNP profiling, this technique is ideal for severely degraded DNA samples.

6. Like the Y chromosome, mtDNA is very stable because it undergoes very little, if any, recombination. Many mitochondria are present in each cell, resulting in a high copy number of mtDNA per cell, which makes mitochondrial profiling especially useful and the technique of choice in situations where samples are small, old, or degraded, which is often the case in catastrophes.

7. A profile probability provides a mathematical probability that a sample of DNA taken at random from a population shares the same DNA profile as another sample. The information needed to calculate this probability is the identities of alleles present in the sample and their frequencies in the population.

8. The FBI maintains the Combined DNA Index System (CODIS), which is a collection of state and federal DNA databases and the analytical tools needed to mine the data. As of January 2019, the database contained more than 18 million DNA profiles, collected from convicted offenders, forensic investigations, and, in some states, those suspected of crimes, as well as from unidentified human remains and missing persons.

9. DNA phenotyping uses statistical analysis of SNP genotypes to predict a person's physical features and ancestry. Law enforcement currently uses this technique to help identify unknown missing persons and to provide leads in cold cases. This technique has not yet been validated for use in court.

10. Many criminal cases do not have DNA evidence or DNA evidence would not be useful. For those cases for which DNA *is* useful, samples can remain unprocessed. Human error—or deliberate human interference—can introduce errors into DNA evidence. Frequently samples from crime scenes are not pure, but instead contain mixtures of DNA from multiple people. In addition, evidence can be degraded and will produce only a partial profile, which can be difficult to interpret.

Discussion Question Answers

1. Generally, natural DNA is contained within cells and is often coupled with various forms of modification (methylation, associated proteins), whereas synthetic DNA is normally free of these factors. Several methods currently exist that can determine methylation status of a DNA sample. Various treatments of DNA with nucleases can often reveal DNA that has been modified.

2. Using your search engine of choice, search for "regulations regarding the collection and storage of DNA samples and profiles." Even without specifying your state of residence, you can find many sites that provide this type of information. Another strategy is to access the National Conference of State Legislatures Web site and navigate to "Welcome to the DNA Laws Database." There, one can select a particular state to review its laws and regulations regarding DNA collection and profiling.

3. To properly defend a client, it would be absolutely critical that the jury understand the limitations of DNA-based evidence. Refer to the answer to Review Question 10 for some of these limitations.

4. Somatic mosaicism and chimerism involve a mixture of cell types that have different origins within one individual. A chimeric individual contains a mixed population of cells; therefore, a DNA sample taken from one tissue site may not match a DNA sample taken from another site. This can lead to a conflicted set of results when it comes to matching an individual's DNA profile to that from a crime scene sample. Taking DNA samples from various sites on an individual might be useful in mitigating such confusion. In addition, in STR DNA profiling, mosaicism might be detectable at the electrophoresis/analysis stage by the presence of additional peaks or peak height imbalances.

Review and Discussion Questions (Special Topics #6): Genetically Modified Foods

Review Question Answers

1. Selective breeding takes advantage of naturally occurring genotypic differences in populations of organisms to generate strains that showed favorable or desirable traits. Genetically modified organisms, by contrast, have been altered using recombinant DNA technology, which allows modification of agriculturally important organisms to be done more rapidly and with greater precision.

2. Genetic engineering allows genetic material to be transferred within and between species and to alter expression levels of genes. A transgenic organism is one that involves the transfer of genetic material *between different species*, whereas the term cisgenic is used in cases where gene transfers occur *within a species*. Currently, most genetically modified (GM) organisms are transgenic; however, this may change as gene editing techniques are increasingly used.

3. In the United States, only about two dozen genetically modified crops are widely in use. The most common are soybeans and maize.

4. *Bacillus thuringiensis* (Bt) produce crystal (Cry) proteins that are toxic to certain orders of insects. When ingested by susceptible insects, the Cry proteins bind to receptors in the gut wall, which leads to a breakdown of the gut membranes and the death of the insect.

5. Some measures include providing high-dose vitamin A supplements and encouraging growth of fresh fruits and vegetables, but success has been limited due to the costs involved. In the 1990s, Golden Rice, a GM crop, was developed to synthesize the vitamin A precursor, beta-carotene, but only modest levels were made. A later version, Golden Rice 2, produces substantially higher levels of beta-carotene. At present, Golden Rice 2 is being tested for safety and efficacy.

6. Golden Rice 2 is the second-generation transgenic rice crop, developed to synthesize beta-carotene. Its production involved the introduction of three genes into the T-DNA region of a Ti plasmid: a bacterial *carotene desaturase* (*crtI*) gene, which is under the control of an endosperm promoter; the maize *phytoene synthase* (*psy*) gene, also under the control of an endosperm promoter; and the bacterial *phosphomannose isomerase* (*pmi*) gene, which is under the control of a constitutive promoter. Researchers transformed established embryonic rice cell cultures and employed a positive selection method by growing plant cells on a mannose-containing medium. Surviving cells (those that expressed the *pmi* gene) were stimulated to form calluses, which were grown into plants. The desired transgenic constructs were verified using the polymerase chain reaction.

7 The biolistic method of gene introduction achieves DNA transfer by coating particles made of heavy metals with the transforming DNA and firing the coated particles at high speed into plant cells using a gene gun. The introduced DNA might migrate into the cell nucleus and integrate into a plant chromosome.

Transformation using *Agrobacterium*-mediated technology uses a genetically engineered Ti plasmid as a vector to carry exogenous DNA into plant cells. This method results in a higher rate of transformation when compared to the biolistic method, since the Ti plasmid can integrate the cloned DNA directly into the plant genome at random sites.

8. In positive selection, conditions are arranged such that only the organism of interest can grow (mannose selection, for example). In negative selection, a condition is arranged that inhibits the growth of organisms that are of no interest (antibiotic resistance, for example).

9. GM foods are transgenic, relying on the introduction of foreign genes to confer new phenotypes upon them. In the case of Golden Rice 2, three enzyme-encoding genes from three different plants were introduced, using a plasmid vector that was also not native to rice. Gene-modified plants, by contrast, are cisgenic and contain no foreign DNA. Their phenotype is changed by altering endogenous genes. In the case of the CRISPR mushroom, a single gene was mutated and rendered inactive. Furthermore, these alterations are small—usually only several nucleotides long—and precise, unlike the random integration of full-length genes required in GM plants.

Discussion Question Answers

1. In many states, bills have been filed that range from banning GM foods to requiring labeling of such foods. To determine the status of such measures in your state, search for "GM food [your state]" on a major search engine. A comprehensive look at the position the United States takes on foods from genetically modified plants can be found at the U.S. Food and Drug Administration Web site (https://www.fda.gov/Food/IngredientsPackagingLabeling/GEPlants/default.htm).

2. Many positions have been taken and bills have been filed in various states to address the question of GM food labeling. Generally, many feel a "right to know" would allow consumers to make educated choices about the food they consume. They would consider it an advantage to be able to judge the safety of a given food if they had information about the possibility that it contains GM components. Others wonder about the usefulness of a GM label if there is little information provided as to how the food has been modified. Of what value would it be to know that food was genetically modified if the science and specifics about the modifications were not included? How much background knowledge would be needed by the consumer to be able to interpret such information?

3. At this point in time there is probably no "correct" answer that can be given. Advocates both for and against GM foods make valid points in their arguments. For example, while there are no reports of negative health effects, most GM foods are not directly consumed by humans. Required animal tests have shown no toxic effects, but these tests are short-term, and animal tests are not always predictive of effects in humans. Some questions to consider: Even if human clinical trials were conducted, would this provide assurance that no one would experience negative effects? If foreign DNA were found in humans, how would we know that it came from GM crops and not from some other source? These are but a few of the issues that face consumers as more and more GM products hit the market.

Review and Discussion Questions (Special Topics #7): Genomics and Precision Medicine

Review Question Answers

1. Pharmacogenomics assesses the effect an individual's entire genome has on his/her drug responses and targets drug development to specific subpopulations of patients with similar profiles. By contrast, pharmacogenetics focuses on how sequence variations in a specific gene affects an individual's response to drugs.

2. Herceptin is used to treat breast cancers that have amplified the *HER-2* gene and overexpress its product, a tyrosine kinase receptor protein. Herceptin acts by binding the extracellular domain of the receptor and prevents signaling that would normally trigger cell proliferation. This inhibition leads to cell-cycle arrest and death of the cancer cell. Herceptin acts only on cancer cells that have amplified *HER-2* genes, so it is important to know the HER-2 status of each tumor. Molecular tests that are conducted include immunohistochemistry, which detects HER-2 receptors on tumor cells, and fluorescence *in situ* hybridization, which assesses the number of *HER-2* genes.

3. Cytochrome P450 is a family of enzymes that are involved in the metabolism of drugs. Certain variants of cytochrome P450 metabolize drugs slowly and can lead to harmful accumulations of a drug. Other variants cause drugs to be eliminated quickly, which can lead to drug ineffectiveness. Some examples are the CYP2D6 protein, which influences the metabolism of approximately 25 percent of all drugs; CYP2C19, a liver enzyme that is responsible for the metabolism of 10–15 percent of drugs; and CYP2C9, a protein that influences the response to warfarin, an anticoagulant drug.

4. Repression of T cells by cancer cells can be indirect. Abnormal expression of MHC molecules allows cancer cells to avoid recognition by antigen-presenting cells, thereby preventing activation of T cells. Cancer cells can also repress T cell activity directly by synthesizing molecules that bind to and repress T cells. Another direct strategy is by taking advantage of the presence of tumor-associated regulatory T cells (T-regs) or tumor-infiltrating cells (macrophages and monocytes), all of which suppress T cell activity.

5. Adoptive cell transfer is an *in vitro* method to dramatically increase the number of lymphocytes that recognize a specific tumor and to reintroduce these cells back into the patient as an antitumor therapy. Tumor-infiltrating lymphocytes (TILs) are removed and grown in petri dishes with tumor cells and growth factors. TILs that kill tumor cells are selected, retested, and grown to high numbers before being reinfused into patients. This treatment has been remarkably successful in clinical trials to treat metastatic melanoma, encouraging use of this method to treat cervical cancer and some blood cancers.

6. Chimeric antigen receptors are genetically engineered proteins that are expressed on T cells and allow them to recognize tumor cells without activation by antigen-presenting cells. The chimeric proteins contain five key domains: a signal peptide, which directs the protein to the cell surface; the variable regions, which recognize and bind a specific antigen; a linker region, which allows the variable domains to position themselves correctly; a transmembrane domain; and the intracellular signaling domain. The protein is made by cloning DNA fragments encoding each domain into a single molecule and introducing this construct into naïve T cells of the patient.

7. Many genes in the genome are not related to cancer, but many are, and those cancer genes should be assayed as to their expressive state. To develop therapies for effective personalized medicine, the activities of those suites of genes specific to a particular cancer must be assessed. In addition, research has shown that gene expression profiles can change with time and circumstances, which will ultimately affect phenotype, including responses to drugs.

8. As of late October 2018, 55,308 tests were described on this Web site, most of which are used diagnostically. One example of single-gene testing occurs for patients with Campomelic dysplasia, a disease characterized by abnormal skeletal growth, cervical spine instability, progressive scoliosis, and hearing loss. The associated gene is *SOX9*, located on the long arm of chromosome 17, at region 24.3. The molecular tests available are (1) analysis for deletions

217

or duplications, using a method called Multiplex Ligation-dependent Probe Amplification (MLPA) and (2) sequencing of the coding region by Sanger sequencing of both strands, looking for gene variants. By exploring the entries on the Web site, you should be able to identify many more examples of single-gene testing.

Discussion Question Answers

1. The use of genomic studies to develop personalized disease treatments provides an ever-expanding promise for the enhancement of human health and welfare. However, at this point in time, genomic information is available for which useful interpretation may be lacking. In other words, one might have information as to a correlation between a genomic profile and a diseased state, but the question of causal relationships may be unanswerable given the present state of knowledge. What does one do with such information? In addition, in some cases, a treatment approach may be obvious, but the treatment itself may not be available. Also, personalized, targeted treatments are often very expensive; how does one afford a treatment if it is not covered by insurance and financial relief is not forthcoming?

2. A number of technical challenges must be overcome. Current methodologies need to be faster, more accurate, and less expensive. In addition, coordinating the storage of and access to the vast amounts of data that will be generated will be daunting. Once the data are generated, scientists and health professionals will need to ensure that all relevant information is linked. In addition, nonmedical or nongenetic information, such as the effects of environment, life style, and epigenetic contributions will need to be included. The gap between data collection and interpretation of complex interactions will need to be closed, as well. This will likely require changing education parameters for medical students and the training of more genetics counsellors and genomics specialists.

3. Because it is presently impossible to ensure database security, even though efforts are most sincere, one might conclude that medical records will not be completely secure. A concerted effort to improve cybersecurity will definitely be needed.

4. At present, genetic discrimination does exist; however, recent developments in health-care laws seek to minimize such discrimination by medical insurance companies and employers through the Genetic Information Nondiscrimination Act (GINA). It remains to be seen whether genetic discrimination in the workplace will continue.